"This book brings hope and help to a lot of people who are suffering needlessly from fears of blood, injections, or medical procedures. It not only explains why these fears are there in the first place, but also gives the reader clear and solid solutions to the problem.

Antony and Watling have done a tremendous job of synthesizing the best available scientific data and presenting it in a straightforward, reader-friendly format. They take the reader step-by-step through the process, showing them why they feel the way they do and how to get better by facing their fears gradually."

—David F. Tolin, Ph.D., director of the Anxiety Disorders Center at The Institute of Living and assistant professor of psychiatry at the University of Connecticut School of Medicine

"Of all phobias, medical fears are the most serious because they can stop people seeking life-saving medical care. Fortunately here is a book that outlines in a clear, stepwise manner a plan to help people with medical phobias. Drawing on the best available scientific knowledge of evidence-based therapies, the authors translate these treatments into a straightforward and potentially life-saving program. In an easy-to-read style, the authors explain where medical fears come from and then what to do about them. For anyone who avoids medical or dental care because of fear or because they may faint, there is no better place to begin treatment than with reading this book and then doing what it says. For psychologists and other mental health professionals, this book provides an excellent workbook to use when working with people suffering from medical phobias."

—Andrew Page, associate professor of
psychology at the University of Western
Australia in Crawley, Australia

OVERCOMING
medical phobias

how to conquer fear
of blood, needles,
doctors, & dentists

Martin M. Antony, PhD
& Mark A. Watling, MD

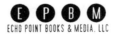

ECHO POINT BOOKS & MEDIA, LLC

Published by Echo Point Books & Media
Brattleboro, Vermont
www.EchoPointBooks.com

Copyright © 2015, 2006 Martin M. Antony and Mark A. Watling
Overcoming Medical Phobias
ISBN: 978-1-62654-351-5 (paperback)
978-1-62654-352-2 (casebound)

Printed and bound in the United States of America

For Aliyana

—M.M.A.

For Mary, Grace, and Sophie

—M.A.W.

contents

acknowledgments

A special thank you to David Grant and Randi McCabe for their assistance in preparing several chapters of this book. We would also like to thank Professor Lars-Göran Öst and others for their pioneering work in developing and researching effective treatments for phobias of blood, needles, and related situations. Finally, we want to express our gratitude to our editors, Catharine Sutker, Heather Mitchener, and Jasmine Star; to Amy Shoup for designing another fantastic cover; and to all the staff at New Harbinger, who are always such a pleasure to work with.

introduction

A hospital is no place to be sick.
> —Samuel Goldwyn (1882–1974)

*Doctors are just the same as lawyers; the only difference
is that lawyers merely rob you, whereas doctors rob and
kill you too.*
> —Anton Chekhov (1860–1904)

Anxiety about visiting doctors and dentists, getting
injections, having or watching surgery, and seeing blood or
having blood drawn are all common in our society. For
example, Dan Piraro (author of the daily syndicated cartoon *Bizarro*) published a cartoon in 1996 depicting a dentist working on a terrified patient. In the background,

through the window of the office, a striped barbershop pole was in view, and the word "barbershop" was written on the outside of the window. The dentist explained to his patient (who had come in for a haircut), "Yes, it does say 'barbershop' out front—when it said 'dental surgeon,' I didn't get nearly as many customers." This cartoon is a nice illustration of just how normal it is to be apprehensive about visiting the dentist.

There are many books available on the general topics of fear, anxiety, and phobias. However, this is the first book that we are aware of that focuses specifically on the topic of medical phobias, fear of blood and needles, and anxiety about going to the dentist. This book is not meant for the person who has only mild levels of anxiety when going to the dentist or doctor. A bit of anxiety is normal in these situations. Rather, the book is meant for people who have more significant levels of anxiety or fear—to the point that the anxiety is bothersome or gets in the way of things that you need or want to do. If you or a family member has significant problems around blood, needles, doctors, or dentists, then this book is for you.

Note that this is not a book about overcoming "health anxiety." If you worry excessively that you may have some serious medical illness, have unrealistic worries about your health, or frequently visit your doctor to check out every little symptom, that's a different type of anxiety problem. To deal with anxiety and worry about your health, we recommend you check out a book by Gordon Asmundson and Steven Taylor (2005) called *It's Not All in*

*Your Head: How Worrying About Your Health Could Be
Making You Sick—and What You Can Do About It.*

how this book is organized

This book contains nine chapters. Chapters 1 and 2 provide general information about the nature and treatment of medical and dental phobias, including a description of these problems and discussion of their prevalence, the impact on those who suffer from these fears, possible causes, and a brief summary of the methods for overcoming these phobias. Chapters 3 and 4 review steps for initially preparing to tackle your fears. Chapters 5, 6, and 7 provide detailed descriptions of proven techniques for overcoming fear related to medical and dental phobias, as well as techniques to combat the tendency to faint, which is often a component of blood and needle fears. After completing the exercises described in these chapters, you should notice a reduction in your anxiety and fear. Chapter 8 is designed to make sure your fear doesn't return in the future. Finally, chapter 9 provides ideas to help family members and friends assist an individual who is trying to cope with anxiety concerning blood, needles, and medical or dental situations. However, we recommend that a helper or interested family members read the entire book, not just chapter 9, in order to better understand the nature and treatment of their loved one's problem.

how to use this book

We recommend that you begin by reading the entire book once, without stopping to complete any of the exercises. This can be done over the course of a few hours. The purpose of the initial reading is to get a general idea of the types of strategies that you will be using when you begin to work on your fear. Next, we recommend that you return to the beginning of the book and begin working through the chapters in more detail, this time completing all recommended exercises. Some chapters can be reviewed very quickly. For example, chapters 1 and 2 contain relatively few exercises, mostly designed to heighten awareness of the causes and symptoms of your own fear. These exercises may take only a few minutes each to complete. Chapters 3 and 4 may take longer to work through, as they require you to develop a detailed treatment plan, including a hierarchy of feared situations that will be used to guide the exposure practices that you'll complete when working through chapter 5.

Several of the other chapters will require more time. For example, chapter 5 describes strategies for directly confronting feared situations, in a safe and controlled way, until they are no longer frightening. This chapter describes exposure therapy—the most important strategy for overcoming a phobia. Strategies such as exposure require repeated practice. Therefore, it may take you several days or even several weeks to work through the techniques described in chapter 5.

If you don't have a history of fainting (or a history of almost fainting) when you get an injection, have blood drawn, or see blood, you can skip chapter 6. However, if you do have a history of fainting in these situations, you should pay close attention to chapter 6 and use the strategies for preventing fainting in conjunction with the exposure strategies described in chapter 5. The strategies described in chapter 7 can also be used at the same time as those reviewed in chapters 5 and 6. The material in chapters 5, 6, and 7 will be relevant during the entire period that you are actively working on conquering your fear. Refer back to these chapters as needed.

Although you will have read chapter 8 early on, during your initial quick review of the book, this chapter should be read again later in the course of your treatment, after you have mastered the exercises described in chapters 5, 6, and 7. It is probably not necessary for you to read chapter 9 again; chapter 9 is designed to be read in detail by any family members or friends who are helping you to work on your fear. Your coverage of this chapter during your initial read of the book should be good enough for your purposes.

obtaining a journal

The strategies described in this book require you to monitor your progress as you go along, and the book is filled with exercises that require you to record various types of information. Therefore, you'll need to pick up some sort of journal or notebook to be used as you work your way through the book. Alternatively, you can record the required information electronically on a computer if you prefer.

is this book likely to help?

The strategies described in this book have been shown in many studies to be effective for treating phobias of needles, blood, dentists, and doctors (for a review, see Antony and Barlow 2002). However, all of the existing studies are based on treatments administered by a therapist. Despite the fact that there are no studies investigating whether treatment for this type of phobia can be administered effectively in a self-help format, there are a few reasons to think that this book is likely to be useful.

First, the self-help treatments described in this book are similar to the therapist-delivered treatments used in studies on blood, needle, medical, and dental phobias (Hellström, Fellenius, and Öst 1996; Moore and Brødsgaard 1994; Öst, Fellenius, and Sterner 1991). In addition, the treatments described in this book tend to work quickly. For example, a number of studies have found that a single session of exposure lasting two to three hours (as described in chapter 5) is enough for many people with blood, needle, and dental phobias to overcome their fear (Hellström, Fellenius, and Öst 1996; Larson et al. 2004; Öst 1989). Finally, although there have been no studies of self-help treatments for medical and dental phobias, there is evidence that some people can benefit from self-help treatments for other types of phobias and anxiety problems (Gould and Clum 1995; Hellström and Öst 1995; Öst, Stridh, and Wolf 1998; Park et al. 2001).

Although these treatments are effective, don't expect that just reading this book will lead to any changes in your fear. To benefit from reading this book, it's important that you practice the exercises and strategies described herein. Also, self-help treatments for anxiety tend to work best when the individual's progress is being monitored by someone else (Febrarro et al. 1999). Therefore, you may want to make a point of involving a family member, close friend, family doctor, or therapist in your treatment. In fact, if your treatment involves exposure to doctors, dentists, or medical procedures, it's going to be difficult to do the treatment without involving one or more health care professionals.

The treatment strategies described in this book are not easy. It's likely that overcoming your fears will first require you to do things that make you very uncomfortable. The good news is that these treatments are effective and they can work relatively quickly. With support from a therapist, doctor, friend, or family member, you should be able to work through the exercises described in this book and experience a dramatic reduction in your fear.

1

about blood, injection, and medical phobias

For as long as she could remember, Lucy was terrified of getting injections. Her fear began as a child, after fainting while getting stitches for a cut on her hand. Over the next few years, she fainted several times during blood tests, vaccinations, and other situations involving needles. As a young adult, she would worry about visits to her doctor for weeks before her appointment. Eventually, she started avoiding doctors completely. She also avoided going to the dentist for fear that she might need a filling or some other procedure requiring numbing. Even watching an injection on television or in a movie was enough to make Lucy feel faint. For years, she dealt with her problem by avoiding the situations she feared. For example, she avoided visiting her husband when he spent a week in the hospital for knee surgery.

Zack was accepted into medical school and was gearing up to start in the fall. There was only one problem: he was terrified of blood. Seeing blood, watching surgery, and even talking about medical procedures made him feel faint. On several occasions he had passed out in these types of situations. Though he was very interested in being a physician, he wasn't sure whether he would be able to start medical school because of his fear.

Randy was diagnosed with a tumor in his pituitary gland. His doctor recommended immediate surgery. Randy's worry about the surgery was manageable—after all, he knew he would be unconscious. However, he was terrified of all the blood work he needed before the surgery, and he was also frightened of the injection he would need to get when being sedated by the anesthesiologist. Randy delayed his surgery for six months before finally getting help for his fear.

Although a mild fear of blood, needles, doctors, or dentists can often be managed without significant interference in a person's life, these three examples illustrate how such fears can cause significant problems for some people. It is the presence of significant distress and impairment that distinguishes a full-blown phobia from an unrealistic fear that isn't really a problem. For a fear to be diagnosed as a *phobia*, it has to be excessive or unrealistic, and it has to bother the person or interfere with his or her functioning in some important way (American Psychiatric Association 1994). This chapter provides an overview of the nature and treatment of blood, needle, medical, and dental phobias.

common features of blood, needle, medical, and dental phobias

Although phobias of blood, needles, doctors, and dentists differ from person to person, there are certain basic features that are common among many people who suffer from these problems. These include characteristic physical and emotional responses, thoughts, and behaviors.

physical and emotional responses

For most phobias, including those of animals, insects, driving, flying, heights, enclosed places, and storms, the most common reaction to the feared object or situation is one of extreme fear or panic, including a wide range of physical symptoms such as a racing or pounding heart, tight muscles, rapid breathing, trembling, sweating, breathlessness, and feeling fidgety. These symptoms are also common in fears of blood, needles, doctors, and dentists. However, a significant number of people with medical phobias respond to their feared situations in a somewhat different way—one that includes fainting.

fainting in blood and needle phobias

For many people with blood and needle phobias, the most common reaction is a two-stage response. First, upon anticipating the situation, they start to experience the common symptoms of fear and anxiety that were mentioned earlier, including an initial increase in heart rate and blood pressure. However, upon actually encountering the situation (for example, when they see blood or get an injection), their heart rate and blood pressure drop very quickly, sometimes leading to fainting (Öst, Sterner, and Lindahl 1984; Page 1994). It is believed that these changes are controlled by the *vagus nerve*, which affects activity in the chest and abdomen. The drop in blood pressure and heart rate is therefore sometimes referred to as *vasovagal syncope*. "Vasovagal" refers to the interaction between blood vessels (vaso) and nerves (vagal), and "syncope" is just a medical term that means fainting. More than half of people with needle phobias and almost three-quarters of people with blood phobias report a history of fainting in the situations they fear (Öst 1992). In contrast, fainting is extremely rare in other types of phobias, including fears of dentists (unless the fear of dentists is a consequence of fearing needles).

It's important to note that for more than a quarter of people with blood phobias and almost half of people with needle phobias, fainting never occurs. In these cases, the fear and avoidance are related to factors other than a fear of fainting (for example, a fear of pain from a needle). Also, about a third of people who faint upon exposure to blood report no fear of blood whatsoever (Kleinknecht and Lenz 1989). So, although fears of blood and fainting often go together, this is not always the case. A person can be afraid despite not fainting, and a person can faint and not be afraid.

It is perfectly normal to experience a drop in blood pressure and heart rate upon exposure to blood, injections, and medical procedures (Schwartz, Adler, and Kaloupek 1987). The problem in blood and needle phobias is that these symptoms are more intense compared to those experienced by the average person. Whereas the average person may experience a slight change in blood pressure or heart rate, the physical changes experienced by someone with a blood phobia are strong enough to cause fainting.

the role of disgust

People who fear blood, injections, and related situations often also have a tendency to be especially sensitive to situations that trigger feelings of disgust (Woody and Teachman 2000). In fact, with the exception of certain animal phobias, fear of blood, injections, and medical procedures are the only phobias known to be associated with an increased tendency to experience disgust. Even people without phobias may experience feelings of disgust when looking at a wound or watching surgery on television, but these feelings are experienced much more strongly by people with phobias of blood and needles. In fact, one study of people with needle phobias found that disgust was the predominant reaction (even stronger than fear) when looking at photos of people getting injections (Tolin et al. 1997).

In addition to experiencing feelings of disgust when confronting blood and needles, there is evidence that people with blood and injection phobias experience a greater than normal amount of disgust when confronted with disgusting images that have nothing to do with their fear (Sawchuk et al. 1997; an example would be watching films depicting maggots). In other words, the increased tendency to feel disgust that sometimes occurs in blood and needle phobias appears to be general, and not just related to situations involving blood and needles.

Studies disagree about whether fainting in blood and needle phobias is most closely related to the emotion of fear versus disgust (Antony and Barlow 2002). The good news is that, regardless of whether your own reaction is primarily one of disgust or fear, treatment is likely to work. Following treatment, you should notice a reduction in both of these unpleasant emotions (Butcher et al. 2003).

exercise: your physical responses

In your journal, describe the most common physical symptoms you experience upon encountering the objects and situations you fear. Do you tend to get a rush of fear or a panicky feeling? If so, what physical sensations tend to be associated with your panic? Do you faint in the situations you fear? What percentage of the time do you actually faint? How long are you typically unconscious when you faint?

phobic thinking

Although emotions such as fear and disgust often seem to come on quickly and automatically when encountering blood, needles, or related situations, many experts believe that these emotions are in fact often triggered by anxious thoughts, predictions, assumptions, and interpretations. In other words, when you start to feel uneasy about going to the doctor or dentist, it may be because you're interpreting the situation as dangerous, or because you're predicting that bad things may happen if you go. For example, if you predict that an injection will hurt, that it will cause you to faint, or that you may get sick from the needle, it's no wonder that you feel anxious.

Anxious thoughts and predictions often occur very quickly and may be outside of your awareness, so your fear seems to occur automatically. In addition, though your thoughts often include predictions about the situation (for example, "the needle will hurt"), they also may include negative predictions about your own reactions to the situation (for example, "if I become too anxious, I will faint, die, or embarrass myself"). Chapter 7 provides a detailed discussion of the role of thoughts in causing or maintaining fear, as well as strategies for changing your anxious thoughts.

---

exercise: your anxious thoughts

In your journal, list any negative thoughts that run through your mind when you think about encountering the objects or situations you fear. List each thought in the form of a prediction about what you fear may happen. Include predictions about the situation itself (for example, "the pain from the dentist's drill will be unmanageable"), as well as predictions about your reactions to the situation (for example, "if I become too anxious, I won't be able to stay and my doctor will think I'm crazy").

phobic behavior

When a person experiences fear, all of the body's resources become focused on doing whatever it takes to reduce the level of fear and to eliminate any perceived threats or dangers. Therefore, the most common behavioral response to a feared situation or object is one of avoidance. If you fear going to the dentist, visiting hospitals, getting injections, having surgery, seeing blood, or getting a physical exam, chances are that you'll try to avoid these situations, sometimes even at great personal risk or cost. Or, if you do enter a feared situation, you may only allow yourself to be exposed to the situation partially. For example, you may go to your family doctor, but then decide not to mention certain symptoms if you believe that talking about these symptoms may lead your doctor to order blood tests.

Avoidance can also be very subtle. For example, you may decide to look away when you get an injection, lie down when you get a blood test, or distract yourself with music at the dentist's office. Avoidance (including subtle forms of avoidance) has advantages and disadvantages. In the short term, avoidance keeps you from feeling uncomfortable. It may also prevent some of the consequences you fear, such as fainting during a blood test. However, in the long term, avoidance may prevent you from getting over your fear, particularly if your fear is unrealistic or exaggerated. This issue will be discussed in more detail in chapter 5.

---

exercise: your anxious behavior

In your journal, list strategies you use to manage your anxiety, avoid feeling fear, or prevent fainting. These strategies may include overt forms of avoidance and escape, or more subtle forms, such as distraction or relying on various safety behaviors designed to make the situation more manageable. (*Safety behaviors* are any actions you take that are designed to protect you from feeling anxious in the situations you fear.)

---

who develops medical and dental phobias?

Fears of blood, injections, and related situations are fairly common. For example, a large study in the United States found that 13.9 percent of people have an extreme fear of blood, and for about a third of these individuals, the fear is severe enough to be considered a phobia (Curtis et al. 1998). In a European study (Fredrikson et al. 1996), 1.6

percent of people were found to have a phobia of injections, 2.1 percent had a phobia of dentists, and 3.3 percent had a phobia of injuries. This study also reported on the differences in prevalence between men and women. Unlike other types of phobias (for example, fears of animals, flying, or enclosed places), in which the prevalence is much higher in women than in men, the prevalence of medical and dental phobias is similar across the sexes.

In our own research (Antony, Brown, and Barlow 1997), we found that fears of blood, injections, and medical situations often begin in childhood (at an average age of 7.93 years). However, we also found that these fears often don't cause significant distress or interference in people's lives for the first few years. In our study, these fears did not reach phobic proportions until an average age of 14.5 years. Generally, other research confirms that these fears tend to begin in childhood or adolescence, on average (Himle et al. 1989; Öst 1987). Of course, there are some people who have had their fear for as long as they can recall, and others who develop their fear later in life.

the impact of medical and dental phobias

For some people, the fear is very focused. For example, we once treated a physician who was terrified of getting an injection himself, though he was comfortable seeing blood, taking blood from his patients, and giving injections to others. We have also seen individuals who are comfortable seeing their own blood (during menstruation or from a nosebleed), but faint at the sight of anyone else's blood. Some people are afraid of only certain types of needle uses (for example, a blood test but not an injection).

For other people, the fear may be more widespread. Fears of blood, needles, surgery, and injury-related situations often go together (Öst 1992), and it is not unusual to fear a wide range of objects and situations having to do with blood, needles, and medical procedures. For example, one study found that 53 percent of people with dental phobias also had a fear of needles, and about 10 percent also had a fear of blood (Poulton et al. 1998).

For many people, a fear of blood, needles, or medical procedures causes only mild impairment. For example, the fear may mean having to look away during certain scenes in a movie or avoiding getting an annual flu shot. However, for others the fear can have serious implications for their health, work, and even relationships. Imagine not being able to visit a spouse or child who is confined to a hospital bed because of a fear of doctors! Even if your fear doesn't cause you serious problems now, phobias of medical procedures sometimes catch up with us. A person with a fear of needles who develops diabetes may risk not performing regular blood tests or not complying with an insulin regimen. Sooner or later, a fear of going to the dentist can lead to serious dental problems because of the lack of regular visits. Or, avoiding all blood work may lead you to miss early signs of an illness, allowing it to become more serious. As we get older, we are confronted with medical situations more and more often. The importance of overcoming your fear will only become greater over time.

Phobias tend to persist unless a person seeks treatment or life circumstances force the person to confront the feared situations. For example, some women with needle phobias naturally overcome their fears during pregnancy because of all the blood work they require. However, for most people, the fear continues until the person makes a conscious decision to overcome it.

overcoming your fears

For most anxiety-related problems, a range of effective treatment options exists, including medications and psychological approaches. In the case of blood, needle, and medical phobias, there are no studies supporting the use of medications as a strategy for overcoming fear over the long term. However, evidence from at least one study indicates that taking an antianxiety medication (for example, lorazepam or diazepam) thirty minutes before dental treatment may help reduce anxiety during the dental procedure (Thom, Sartory, and Jöhren 2000).

For people who have a history of fainting, we recommend against the use of antianxiety medications because they are unlikely to help with the fainting response. In fact, they may actually increase the likelihood of fainting by reducing your heart rate or blood pressure even more than is typically the case during vasovagal syncope. Because of the overall lack of evidence supporting medications for blood, needle, medical, and dental phobias, this book will focus more on psychological approaches.

People use many different approaches to deal with psychological and emotional challenges. Examples include seeking support from friends, dietary changes, prayer, "talk therapy," hypnosis, and biofeedback. However, this book will focus only on strategies that have been researched extensively for dealing with phobias. Specifically, we'll focus on techniques that together are often referred to as cognitive and behavioral strategies (the word "cognitive" simply refers to the process of thinking). These include strategies involving changing anxious behaviors, strategies for managing physical symptoms (such as heightened arousal or faintness), and strategies for changing anxious thinking.

exposure-based strategies

Exposure is one of the most powerful strategies for overcoming fear. In fact, it is widely believed that most people don't overcome their phobias without some sort of exposure to the situations they fear. Essentially, exposure involves gradually confronting the feared objects or situations until you are no longer afraid. Numerous studies have confirmed that exposure is effective for overcoming phobias of blood, needles, dentists, and related situations (Antony and Barlow 2002). Exposure is the key strategy used in this book, and we'll discuss it at length in chapter 5.

relaxation-based strategies

Relaxation-based strategies may be useful under certain circumstances, particularly as an add-on to exposure. Specifically, techniques involving imagery, muscle relaxation, or learning to slow down your breathing may help to reduce your anxiety at the doctor's or dentist's office (Jerremalm, Jansson, and Öst 1986; Öst, Sterner, and Fellenius 1989). This book doesn't provide detailed coverage of relaxation-based strategies. If you're interested in learning more about relaxation-based techniques, check out the latest edition of *The Relaxation and Stress Reduction Workbook* (Davis, Eshelman, and McKay 2000).

applied muscle tension

Applied muscle tension is a variation of exposure therapy that combines exposure with muscle tension exercises designed to temporarily increase blood pressure and prevent fainting. This technique is described in detail in chapter 6. If your anxiety is associated with fainting, this is probably the strategy that you'll want to focus on most. The exposure exercises will help reduce your fear and the tension exercises will help prevent fainting along the way (Hellström, Fellenius, and Öst 1996; Öst, Fellenius, and Sterner 1991).

cognitive strategies

In most cases, studies on the treatment of blood and needle phobias have focused mostly on behavioral strategies such as exposure and applied tension. In contrast, studies on the treatment of dental phobias have included a wider range of strategies, including techniques for challenging anxious thinking and replacing negative thoughts with more realistic interpretations and predictions. Treatments that include both behavioral and cognitive elements appear to be useful, particularly for dental phobias (de Jongh et al. 1995; Getka and Glass 1992; Jerremalm, Jansson, and Öst 1986). These strategies are discussed in chapter 7.

summary

This chapter provided an overview of the nature and treatment of blood, needle, medical, and dental phobias. These fears tend to begin in childhood or adolescence, and they occur frequently in both males and females. Though the problem is often associated with typical fear symptoms such as a racing heart and breathlessness, it is unique in that fainting is also a common occurrence, particularly among those with blood and needle phobias. In addition to the experience of fear, the emotion of disgust is also a common feature of these phobias. Negative predictions are thought to contribute to the experience of fear and disgust, and behaviors such as avoidance help to maintain the phobia over time.

The most important component of any effective treatment for these phobias is exposure to the feared objects or situations. Learning to tense all the muscles of the body in order to temporarily raise blood pressure and prevent fainting is very useful in cases where the phobia is associated with fainting. Finally, relaxation exercises and learning to replace anxious thinking with more realistic thinking may be useful additions to exposure therapy.

what causes blood, injection, and medical phobias?

People like to understand the causes of their problems. After all, how can you overcome a problem without understanding the cause? Knowing the cause can help you to select the best treatment, right? Well, that may be true, sometimes, sort of. In reality, the relationship between the cause of a problem and the ideal treatment is often not so clear-cut.

Before going any further, let's distinguish between two types of causes—*initial causes* and *maintaining factors*. Initial causes are those factors that originally triggered the problem, whereas maintaining factors are those variables responsible for keeping the problem active over time. Often, the factors that keep a problem going are not the same as those that initially triggered the problem. Examples of experiences that may have initially triggered your fear include getting a painful injection, fainting during a blood test, or having a bad experience at the dentist's. Examples of factors that may maintain your fear currently include the tendency to avoid feared situations, to rely on safety behaviors, and to misinterpret the situation as dangerous. With respect to phobias, it appears to be most important to understand and change the variables that maintain your fear now. Understanding the original causes matters less, at least from the perspective of overcoming the problem.

There are lots of examples in medicine of treatments that work regardless of how the illness initially began. For example, in order to treat a broken leg, it isn't important to know exactly how the injury occurred. Whether the broken leg was a result of skiing, falling down stairs, or playing football is irrelevant when it comes to deciding how to treat it. It's only important to understand the factors that might prevent it from healing properly (for example, the type of fracture).

Strategies for understanding and changing the thoughts and behaviors that contribute to the maintenance of your fear are discussed later in the book. In this chapter, we focus instead on the factors that may have initially contributed to the development of your fear. Don't worry if you can't remember how your fear began. The treatments described in this book are likely to be useful regardless of the initial cause (Öst 1985).

experiences that contribute to fear

Psychologist S. Rachman (1977) noted three different pathways by which we learn to develop fear: direct personal experience, learning through observation, and learning through information or instruction. Each of these pathways is described below.

direct personal experiences

For many people, phobias seem to begin after they directly experience a negative event involving the object or situation. Here are a few examples of direct personal experiences that may contribute to a fear of blood, needles, doctors, or dentists:

◊ Suffering discomfort while donating blood (for example, experiencing bruising or pain from the technician not being able to find an appropriate vein)

◊ Fainting while getting an injection

◊ Experiencing pain during a dental treatment

learning through observation

For some people, fear is learned by watching someone else be afraid or have a negative experience in a situation. Here are some examples of observational learning:

◊   Growing up with parents who are terrified of doctors and learning to have the same fear by watching them be afraid

◊   Seeing someone faint during a blood test

◊   Observing an older brother cry when he gets an injection as a child

learning through information or instruction

We are continually exposed to information about all sorts of threats in the world. Our parents and teachers warn us of what might happen if we're not careful, our friends tell us of terrible things they've heard about, and the media (including newspapers, television, and books) often exaggerate certain dangers in the world (Glassner 1999). Covers of the world's leading news magazines warn us of the risks associated with terrorism, shark attacks, child abductions, flying in airplanes, crime, road rage, killer diseases, earthquakes, and other threats. In fact, there are a number of recent books devoted exclusively to warning people about the "dangers" they face in everyday life, such as these:

Be Safe! Simple Strategies for Death-Free Living (Heckscher 2004)

Risk! A Practical Guide for Deciding What's Really Safe and What's Really Dangerous in the World Around You (Ropeik and Gray 2002)

*100 Most Dangerous Things in Everyday Life and
What You Can Do About Them* (Lee 2004)

It's no wonder people are worried!

Here are just a few examples of the type of information and instruction that can contribute to a fear of
blood, needles, doctors, dentists, or related situations:

- ◊ Being told by others how painful dental treatment can be

- ◊ Reading a news story about someone getting
  AIDS from a dirty needle

- ◊ Being told by a nurse to look away just before
  getting an injection

- ◊ Reading a magazine article about mistakes that
  can happen during surgery

research on the effects of experience on fear

It's all well and good to discuss the role of experience from a theoretical perspective, but what does the
research actually say about the effects of these experiences on fear? Do people actually develop their fears
through these three pathways?

A number of studies investigating the onset of
blood, needle, and dental fears all tend to find the same
thing (Kendler, Myers, and Prescott 2002; Kleinknecht
1994; Öst 1991; Öst and Hugdahl 1985; Townend,
Dimigen, and Fung 2000). Based on responses from

people who suffer from these fears, direct personal experiences appear to be the most common pathway to developing fear, with between half and three-quarters of people with blood, needle, and dental phobias reporting this type of onset. In contrast, only between 15 and 20 percent of people report learning their fear through observation, and considerably fewer than 10 percent report learning their fear through instruction or information. Between 15 and 40 percent of people don't remember how their fear began. If you are one of those people, you're in good company.

Of course, the factors people believe caused their fear and the factors that actually caused it may be very different. When it comes to trying to understand the causes of phobias, researchers are limited by the accuracy of people's reports about events that often have occurred in the distant past. Also, just because people report having had these experiences doesn't necessarily mean these experiences caused the fear. It's possible that other factors contributed to the fear, and that the fear might have developed regardless of the person's experience.

other factors that may play a role

As mentioned earlier, a significant percentage of people with phobias don't recall a specific event triggering their fear. Also, many people have negative experiences and yet don't develop fears, suggesting that factors other than negative experiences may be important. Genetics, personality, and frequency of exposure are three potential factors in the development of phobias.

genetic factors

For decades, it's been known that phobias run in families. However, knowing this doesn't shed much light on whether the transmission of phobias is due to genetic factors or learning. After all, we usually share experiences with our families, as well as sharing our genetic makeup. A young boy growing up with a mother who is terrified of needles may learn to fear needles by watching his mother, but he may also inherit some of the genes that contribute to the fear. In addition to simply studying the prevalence of phobias among family members, researchers have developed a number of other strategies to better separate out the effects of genetics versus environment.

To really understand the relative contributions of genetics and environment, scientists often study twins. Identical twins (also called *monozygotic twins*) are genetically 100 percent identical, whereas fraternal twins are on average 50 percent identical, just like any other pair of siblings. By examining the relative prevalence of phobias in fraternal versus identical twins of people known to have a phobia, researchers have been able to estimate the extent to which genetic factors contribute to the transmission of phobias across family members.

A large number of studies have now shown that genetic factors play a role in the transmission of phobias in general (Hettema, Neale, and Kendler 2001; Kendler Karkowski, and Prescott 1999), and for blood and injection phobias in particular (Page and Martin 1998). Though some studies suggest that the impact of environment is relatively small (Kendler, Myers, and Prescott 2002; Neale et al. 1994), other research suggests a much larger role for environmental factors (Skre et al. 1993). It's impossible to know for any one individual whether genetics or experience is the largest contributor to the person's fear. In many cases, it may be a combination of these factors that ultimately determines who develops a phobia and who doesn't.

Even if your biological makeup ultimately determined the development of your phobia, psychological methods can still be used to overcome the fear. Changes in behavior can certainly influence a person's biology. For example, if you're genetically predisposed to be obese, develop heart disease, or drink too much alcohol, your behavior can still have an impact on whether your genetic tendency will end up being expressed. Having a genetic predisposition to being fearful simply means that it may be harder for you to reach a point of being nonfearful than it might be for someone else. Regardless of the extent to which genetics has contributed to your fear, the strategies described in this book are likely to be helpful as you work toward overcoming the fear. Success rates for treating these phobias behaviorally tend to be very high.

personality factors

In addition to our learning experiences and genetic makeup, general personality styles may contribute to the development of fear. Of course, personality is influenced by experiences and genetics, so in a way this is not really separate from those variables. The point here is that people who generally have an anxious style of responding to their environment may be more at risk for developing phobias than those who have a less anxious personality style. For example, someone who is generally not especially anxious or worried may be less likely to respond with fear to a negative experience at the dentist's than someone who tends to be more anxious. From a research perspective, little is known about the contribution of personality factors to the development of blood, needle, and medical phobias. The notion that personality style may play a role is nothing more than speculation at this point.

frequency of exposure

Another factor that may influence the development of fear is the amount of exposure a person has to the object or situation. For example, a child who grows up with a diabetic parent requiring daily insulin injections would likely be exposed to injections on a regular basis. This regular exposure might protect the child from developing a needle phobia, compared to an otherwise similar child who hasn't had much exposure to needles while growing up. In other words, regular exposure to blood, needles, doctors, and dentists may protect people from developing medical phobias even if they later have a negative experience in one of these situations.

You have probably heard the old saying that if you fall off a horse, you need to get right back on to prevent fear from setting in. The same is true of many other negative experiences. People who avoid doctors or dentists after experiencing a negative event (for example, a painful needle) may be more likely to develop fear than people who force themselves back into the situation despite the negative experience.

---

exercise: where did your fear come from?

In your journal, list any experiences that may have contributed to your fear. Did you experience some negative event that contributed to the onset of your fear or that led to a worsening of your fear? Can you think of anyone from whom you may have learned your fear? Can you think of anything you've read, heard, or seen that may have led to the development or worsening of your fear? Are there others in your family who have the same fear as you? To what extent does a fear of blood, needles, hospitals, doctors, or dentists run in your family? If you tend to faint in these situations, do others in your family have a similar reaction?

---

summary

This chapter reviewed some of the factors believed to contribute to the development of phobias concerning blood, needles, and medical situations. Various negative experiences, including traumatic events, observing others who are frightened, and coming across negative information about the situation, may contribute to a person's fear. Genetics is also thought to play a role. Factors such as personality and previous exposure to the situation may moderate the influences of genetics and negative learning experiences.

3

developing a hierarchy

One of the most important steps in getting over any fear is confronting it directly. But facing a fear head-on can be quite overwhelming and may even feel impossible given where your fear is at now. As you read this, it may seem as though you'll never be able to go to the dentist, see your doctor, or have blood taken. But there is a way you can do this; it involves taking many small steps toward your goal, rather than trying to do it in one big step.

Suppose you have a friend who is scared of dogs. It may seem obvious to you that in order for your friend to combat her fear, eventually she would have to come into contact with a dog. But she wouldn't have to start by going up to the biggest, scariest dog in the neighborhood. That could be overwhelming even for someone who isn't afraid of dogs. Instead, you might suggest that she start off with a less fearful situation, like looking at a video of a dog or perhaps looking at a small live dog from a reasonable distance. Once she gets used to that initial practice, you might suggest that she get closer to the small dog, and once she gets used to that, you might suggest that she get very close and eventually even try petting the dog.

It's common sense to take small steps to reach your goal. We do this all the time in our day-to-day lives. Think about the small steps taken in learning to drive, learning a new sport, or learning to play a musical instrument. You wouldn't suggest that a person who wants to run a marathon do a full marathon as his or her first-ever run. By taking small steps, you stand a better chance of being successful. And success at each small step will bring you closer to your ultimate goal.

A list of small steps aimed at helping you reach your ultimate goal is called an *exposure hierarchy*. This is a list of situations you plan to expose yourself to, recorded in order of difficulty, or in order of how anxious or fearful they make you feel. The top item represents the ultimate goal, or the most difficult item. Each item represents something you'd like to be able to do if not for your fear.

Each situation is assigned a fear rating ranging from 0 to 100, representing the level of fear that the situation is likely to cause. A rating of 100 means the maximum fear you can imagine experiencing, and a rating of 0 means no fear at all. A rating of 50 refers to a moderate level of fear. Your ratings can be any number between 0 and 100. These ratings are sometimes called SUDS scores (SUDS stands for "subjective unit of distress scale"). This rating of fear is subjective because different people respond to particular situations with different levels of fear.

If your primary emotion upon encountering the situation is something other than fear (for example, disgust), you can use your ratings to measure that emotion instead. Keep that in mind as you develop your hierarchy. The remainder of this chapter will help you develop your own individualized exposure hierarchy for your particular fear of blood, doctors, dentists, or needles. Sample hierarchies are provided at the end of the chapter.

generating your hierarchy

Developing a hierarchy involves five main steps:

1. Generating a list of feared situations

2. Listing the variables that affect your fear level for each situation

3. Combining your initial list with the moderating variables in order to generate a list of more detailed items

4. Assigning a fear rating to each item

5. Refining the hierarchy

We'll now discuss each of these steps in more detail. We recommend that you complete the exercises described in each step as you read through them. (If this is your quick, initial reading of the book, you can put this off until you come back to it during your more detailed reading.)

step 1: generate an initial list of feared situations

If you're afraid of needles and injections, think of all of the various situations in which you might confront this fear. It might help to think of the activities, situations, and objects that you presently avoid because of your fear. Think of the things you'd like to be able to do but can't because of your fear. Think of the things that you can do, but only with tremendous anxiety or fear. Think of the specifics that cause you to be scared in the situation: is it the sight of blood, is it the smell of a hospital, is it the sight of a needle, is it the sound of a dentist's drill? Here are some examples of feared situations for a person with a needle phobia:

◊   Watching a news story about vaccinations

◊   Looking at a picture of a needle

◊   Watching a documentary about operations

◊   Smelling rubbing alcohol

◊   Holding a needle

◊   Watching someone have blood taken

◊   Watching someone get an injection

◊   Having blood taken

◊   Getting a flu shot

For someone with a fear of doctors and hospitals, the list might include situations such as these:

◆   Looking at pictures of doctors

◆   Watching a TV show about doctors (for example, *ER*)

◆   Watching a documentary on plastic surgery

◆   Walking through a hospital corridor

◆   Eating in a hospital cafeteria

◆   Sitting in a family doctor's waiting room

◆   Sitting in a hospital waiting room

◆   Setting up an appointment with a family doctor

◆   Having a physical exam by a family doctor

◆   Getting a flu shot

◆   Having blood taken

◆   Having minor surgery (for example, having a cyst, wart, or mole removed)

exercise: making your list of situations

In your journal, list the objects or situations that you fear. At this stage, list as many items as you can think of, including items from a wide range of difficulty levels. In other words, include items that generate mild, moderate, and severe levels of fear. If an item seems so scary that you can't even imagine doing it, make sure you still include it on the list!

step 2: list the variables that affect your fear level in these situations

Here are some examples of variables that may moderate or affect your fear:

◊   The size of the needle

◊   The personality of your doctor or dentist

◊   Your relationship with the doctor or dentist (for example, how well you know him or her)

◊   The environment in which the exposure occurs (for example, the size or temperature of the room)

◊   Whether you're lying down or sitting up

◊   Whether you're alone or with someone else

◊   Whether you're looking at a color picture or a black and white picture (if you're looking at a photo of a surgical procedure)

◊   The type of procedure being done (for example, a dental cleaning versus a filling)

◊   The time of day

◊   What you're feeling at the time of the exposure (fatigue, hunger, pain)

◊   Your focus of attention (for example, looking at the needle versus looking away)

◊   How the blood is displayed—for example, in a
     tube, in a bag, or exposed on a cut (for a blood
     phobia exposure involving looking at blood)

◊   Distance from the feared object

---

exercise: listing the variables
that affect your fear

In your journal, list the variables that affect the level of
fear, anxiety, or discomfort you experience in the situations you listed in step 1.

---

step 3: incorporate the information in
steps 1 and 2 to generate a list of
detailed hierarchy items

The purpose of this step is to create a list of items
that incorporate both the feared situation (from step 1)
and the variables that affect your fear level in the situation (from step 2). The more detail you include, the
better. Here are some examples of hierarchy items that
are not detailed enough and improved items with greater
detail. These examples will help you to generate items
with sufficient detail:

Original item: Go to the doctor.

Improved item: Go to a female doctor for a full physical.

Original item: Go to the dentist.

Improved item: Get my teeth checked and cleaned by a dentist I have never met.

Original item: Have blood drawn.

Improved item: Have one tube of blood drawn by an experienced technician while sitting up and looking away, with my boyfriend present.

Note that you can split an item to make several new items. For example, an item involving a needle can be turned into three items of varying difficulty by changing the specific details in the situation:

1. **A very difficult item:** Have three tubes of blood drawn by an unknown technician while sitting up and looking at the needle, alone.

2. **A moderately difficult item:** Have three tubes of blood drawn by a familiar technician while sitting up and looking away, with my boyfriend present.

3. **A less difficult item:** Have one tube of blood drawn by a familiar technician while lying down and looking away, with my boyfriend present.

---

exercise: making a list of hierarchy items

In your journal, develop a list of more detailed hierarchy items, taking into account the information from steps 1 and 2. Be as specific as you can for each item. Try to include situations to which you can expose yourself fairly easily (albeit with extreme fear). In other words, don't include items like "have triple bypass surgery" unless you actually want or need to have that procedure done. Also, try to include a number of items that can be repeated. As you'll learn in chapter 5, exposure works best when repeated frequently. Finally, aim to have a completed list of between ten and fifteen items.

step 4: assign a fear rating to each of the items listed in step 3

Step 4 involves assigning a fear rating to each item generated in step 3. Think to yourself, "If I were to face this situation right now, how much fear would I have?"

exercise: putting your items in order

In your journal, rate your fear or discomfort for each item on a scale of 0 to 100 and write that number beside the item. Again, 0 means no fear at all, and 100 refers to the most fear you have ever experienced. Be honest with yourself.

Now rewrite your hierarchy items in order of the fear ratings associated with each one, with the highest-scored item (closest to 100) at the top of the list, and the lowest-scored item at the bottom of the list. You have now completed the first draft of your exposure hierarchy.

step 5: refine your hierarchy

Take a close look at the hierarchy you developed in step 4. Is there a reasonable spread of fear ratings? Ideally, you want about ten to fifteen items that cross over a range of difficulty levels. If you have too many items with high fear ratings, think again about the variables you could change in order to make some items less difficult (changing the situation in some way, for example, standing farther away or completing the exposure with a loved one present). If you don't have enough items in the higher range, try to add some more challenging items or think of ways to modify one of the easier exposures to make it slightly more difficult.

exercise: refining your hierarchy

In your journal, make any needed modifications to your hierarchy so that you have ten to fifteen items ranging from not too difficult (for example, a rating of 30) at the bottom, to very difficult (for example, a rating of 90 or 100) at the top. Note that this isn't your last chance to make changes to your hierarchy. You can continue to add, delete, or modify items throughout the course of your treatment.

sample hierarchies

To assist you in the final steps of developing an individualized hierarchy that will guide you through the exposure
practices described in chapter 5, here are examples of hierarchies for fears of injections, dentists, blood, and doctors
and hospitals.

Sample Exposure Hierarchy for Fear of Injections		
Item	Description	Fear Rating (0–100)
1	Have blood taken at a hospital lab	100
2	Hold a needle while watching someone else having blood taken	90
3	Hold a needle while watching a video of someone having blood taken	85
4	Watch a video of someone having a blood test after I've hyperventilated (breathed quickly) for sixty seconds	80
5	Hold a needle while smelling an alcohol swab	75
6	Have a tourniquet placed on my arm and press a needle against my skin	70
7	Press a needle against my skin with no tourniquet	65
8	Hold a needle with the cap off	50
9	Hold a needle with the cap on	40
10	Hold a syringe without a needle attached	30

	Sample Exposure Hierarchy for Fear of Dentists	
Item	Description	Fear Rating (0–100)
1	Get a tooth filled by a dentist, including a needle and drilling	100
2	Go to dentist for a full cleaning and X-rays, and listen to the sound of a dentist's drill in the background several times during the procedure	95
3	Go to dentist for a full cleaning and X-rays, without listening to the dentist's drill	85
4	Go to a dentist for a checkup (with X-rays), but no cleaning	75
5	Sit in a dentist's chair, no work being done	65
6	Watch a friend have dental work done	60
7	Sit in a dental office waiting room	50
8	Hold a dental instrument while watching a dental video	50
9	Watch a video of a dental cleaning without holding anything	45
10	Hold a dental instrument	35

Item	Description	Fear Rating (0–100)
	**Sample Exposure Hierarchy for Fear of Blood**	
1	Have a blood test, with three vials of blood taken	100
2	Watch someone else have three vials of blood drawn	100
3	Watch a detailed surgery video	90
4	Prick my finger and squeeze out blood	90
5	Watch someone else prick a finger and squeeze out blood	80
6	Watch a video of someone having blood drawn	75
7	Hold a jar containing cow's blood from a roast or steak	60
8	Place fake blood on my daughter's finger and look at it while imagining it's real	50
9	Go to the butcher's counter at a grocery store	40
10	Hold a raw steak	35

Sample Exposure Hierarchy for Fear of Doctors and Hospitals		
Item	**Description**	**Fear Rating (0–100)**
1	See an unfamiliar family doctor for an examination	100
2	See my own family doctor for a physical examination	90
3	See my own family doctor about minor symptoms (for example, a chest cold or back pain), without a full physical examination	75
4	Sit in a hospital waiting room alone	75
5	Sit in a hospital waiting room with my wife	65
6	Have my blood pressure taken by a nurse	65
7	Have my blood pressure taken by a friend	50
8	Walk through the corridor of a hospital	40
9	Watch a hospital TV show, like *ER*	40
10	Go to a medical supply store	35

summary

Before you can begin to use the exposure strategies discussed in chapter 5, it's important to develop an exposure hierarchy—a list of feared situations, arranged from not too difficult (at the bottom) to very difficult (at the top). The hierarchy is like a road map, used to guide the particular steps taken as you gradually begin to confront your fears. Exposure begins at the bottom of the hierarchy and progresses to the higher items. Remember, the hierarchy you developed in this chapter is not written in stone. It is meant to be changed and modified as you proceed through your treatment, as new ideas occur to you, or as you learn more about yourself and your phobia.

4

preparing for treatment

In the last chapter, you learned that treating a phobia requires confronting your fear in a controlled, methodical way by using an exposure hierarchy, and you developed a hierarchy for your own fear. Soon, it will be time to put your exposure plan into action. This may be one of the most difficult parts of treatment, but it is also one of the most rewarding. In chapter 5, you'll confront situations that will probably be very anxiety provoking, which means you may have to really push yourself at times. You may feel discouraged during some practices because your fear seems so strong. It will be important to recognize that "difficult" does not equal "impossible." The discomfort you feel when confronting your fear will be temporary, but the benefits will last a lifetime.

Motivating yourself to work your way up your hierarchy can be difficult. Therefore, it's important to remind yourself why you're doing this. In fact, it may be helpful to make a list of what you stand to gain by facing your fear and overcoming it.

exercise: making a list of reasons to overcome your fear

Take some time right now to think about ways you can keep motivated. Consider how different your life will be once you're over this fear. How will your life be improved? How will the lives of others who are important to you (friends, family, coworkers, and so on) be improved if you get over your fear? Consider other difficult life challenges you've faced successfully and remember how you felt afterward. As you think of various benefits of overcoming your fear, record them on a piece of paper. Keep the list in a prominent place (perhaps on the fridge) to remind yourself why you're doing this.

including a helper in your treatment

Including a helper in your treatment will make it much easier to work through your hierarchy. Your helper may be a good friend or a close family member. Or, it can be a professional therapist (we'll return to the issue of finding a therapist shortly). The ideal helper is someone who is patient, supportive, and familiar with your fear. Your helper should be someone with whom you won't be shy about sharing the many aspects of your phobia, and someone who won't make fun of your fear. A helper should not have the same fear that you're working on (although a helper who has had the same fear in the past and has overcome it may be great).

Including a helper provides a number of advantages. A helper can provide much-needed encouragement. There may be times when you feel like giving up or when you question whether you can do the exposures; a helper can give you the support you might need at those difficult times. A helper can also aid in collecting materials needed for exposure exercises. A helper can preview potential exposure materials for you (such as pictures or videos or anxiety-provoking locations) to help determine their appropriateness at various stages of your therapy. It would be difficult for you to do this yourself. A helper will be able to assist during actual exposure exercises. For example, if you're afraid of having blood drawn, a helper may allow you to watch while his or her blood is drawn as one of your exposures. In this way, a helper can model nonfearful coping behavior during exposures. It's important for your helper to be educated with respect to what's involved in behavior therapy for a specific phobia, so if you do choose to have a helper, it would be great for that person to read this entire book as well. Chapter 9 is especially written for your helper (though you are encouraged to read it too).

If you can't find a helper, you have a few other options. You could enlist the help of a professional, or you can proceed on your own. If you do proceed on your own and you encounter difficulties along the way, you can still consider getting professional help at that point.

finding a therapist

A professional therapist can provide support and help ensure that you're completing the necessary exercises to maximize your chances of success. A professional can offer advice to help you refine your hierarchy or brainstorm with you to find strategies for translating your hierarchy items into real-life practices. A professional therapist (particularly one who specializes in the treatment of anxiety and phobias) may have experience treating many people with problems similar to yours. An experienced therapist will know how to help you face your fear successfully and may be able to help you to avoid some of the obstacles that may arise along the way.

A particular advantage of working with a professional on medical phobias is that the therapist may be able to provide access to specific situations and exposure opportunities that might otherwise be unavailable to you. For example, he or she may have access to medical equipment, colleagues who work in medical or dental settings, or other materials that would normally be hard to come by. A therapist who has treated many people with a phobia similar to yours may already have a supply of some of the more common materials you'll need for exposures. Committing to meeting with a professional may also help motivate you to keep going with your treatment even on days when you just don't feel like it, just as meeting with a personal trainer can make it easier to stick to a fitness plan. If you're going to seek the help of a professional, these are some questions you would want to ask a potential therapist:

◊ What is your professional training? (Ideally, you want a therapist who has professional training in mental health through an advanced degree, such as an MD or Ph.D., or a practitioner with other training, such as a clinical social worker or a master's level therapist.)

◊ Do you have experience treating anxiety disorders? (You want someone experienced in treating phobias and other anxiety problems.)

◊ Where did you learn to treat anxiety disorders? (Ideally, the therapist should have trained at a specialized anxiety clinic or through an academic or university training program.)

◊ Are you experienced in cognitive behavioral therapy (CBT)? (This kind of therapy is also sometimes called "exposure therapy" or "behavior therapy.") Ideally, this is the kind of approach you want your therapist to take in helping to treat your phobia. Be cautious about therapists who recommend another approach or who recommend a blended approach to treatment. Cognitive behavioral therapy (especially exposure) is currently the only treatment proven to be effective for treating blood, needle, medical, and dental phobias.

Remember, you have to be comfortable with the therapist you choose. You may have to interview a few potential therapists before you find one who's the right match for you.

Here are a few suggestions on how to locate a therapist:

- ◊ The Anxiety Disorders Association of America (ADAA) can be accessed through the Internet (www.adaa.org) or by phone (240-485-1001). This organization has an up-to-date list of professionals throughout North America who are experienced in treating phobias. They can also put you in contact with similar associations around the world, including the Anxiety Disorders Association of Canada (www.anxietycanada.ca), for example.

- ◊ Other professional associations may be able to provide you with information about appropriate professionals in your area. The Association for Behavioral and Cognitive Therapies (previously known as the Association for Advancement of Behavior Therapy, www.aabt.org) is one example.

- ◊ Your family doctor or other health care providers may be able to recommend therapists who specialize in treating anxiety disorders. If you have a fear of dentists, your dentist or dental hygienist may be aware of a professional who can help.

◊   You may want to look in the yellow pages under "psychologists," "psychiatrists," or "psychotherapists" to find someone in your area. Remember to look for someone who advertises themselves as a cognitive behavioral therapist with experience in treating anxiety disorders.

Once you've located a therapist, you could consider taking this book to one of your first appointments. This book could serve as a template for you and your therapist to follow as you confront your phobia.

finding the items you need for exposure

To put your plan into action and conduct exposure practices using the hierarchy you developed in chapter 3, you're going to need to locate certain items, objects, pictures, or situations. Here are some specific suggestions for where to find the materials and situations you need, organized by type of phobia.

exposure ideas for medical phobias

Letting your family doctor know that you're working on overcoming your fear may be a good place to start. Your doctor may be able to supply you with items that you can use in your exposures. He or she may also let you sit in the waiting room as an exposure, or even sit in one of the examination rooms when it isn't being used. The following examples of images, activities, objects, and situations may be useful to consider as you plan your exposure practices. As you read through these examples, think about which are relevant to your own fear.

medical images, photos, and videos

There are many movies and TV shows these days with medical themes. Movies such as *The Doctor*, *Patch Adams*, *Vital Signs*, and *Flatliners* all have great medical scenes. Have a look at your local video rental store. Ask store employees if they can suggest any good movies with medical themes. Talk to your friends and family to see if they have any suggestions. If you find a movie with a good medical scene, watch that particular scene repeatedly. Medical-themed television shows are another great resource. Consider taping an episode of *ER* or TLC's *The Operation*. You can then repeatedly expose yourself to various scenes once they're on tape.

On the Internet, search Google's images site (http://images.google.com) using keywords such as "doctors," "surgery," or "operations" for good medical images. Medical journals or textbooks (found in hospital libraries) and medical teaching videos (available at medical school libraries or on the Internet) could be other good items to have a look at.

medical tools and instruments

Items such as reflex hammers, stethoscopes, otoscopes (an instrument for looking in ears), cotton balls, tongue depressors, blood pressure cuffs, and doctors' white coats can be found in drugstores or medical supply stores. Most cities have a medical uniform supply store that sells hospital scrubs, lab coats, and nurses' uniforms. Your family doctor may be able to provide items that are harder to come by, such as IVs, IV bags, blood collecting equipment, needles, and so on. Syringes and needles can be purchased at a pharmacy. Pharmacies also often have in-store blood pressure cuffs for customers to use.

medical settings

Medical settings such as a doctor's office, doctor's waiting room, surgical waiting area, hospital lobby, hospital cafeteria, hospital corridor, or emergency room waiting area are all available in most communities. Look into the hospitals in your community (or have your helper scout them out for you). Your doctor may also be helpful in suggesting locations that may be available to you. And, because people with medical phobias often fear the smell of a doctor's office, you could use rubbing alcohol to create this smell in other settings.

exposure ideas for dental phobias

For starters, your dentist may be a great resource. If you let your dentist or dental hygienist know that you have a fear of dentists, he or she may be more than happy to allow you to sit in a dental chair without getting work done, or to have work done in a very gradual way. Or, they may lend you dental models or teaching videos that you can use for your exposures. Dentists are aware that many people have a fear of dental treatment, and they often want to do what they can to help people overcome their fear. In fact, some dentists specialize in treating patients with dental phobias. Here are some ideas on how to find items or situations that may be useful for your exposure practices.

dental images, photos, and videos

Unfortunately, many movies and TV shows portray dentists in very negative and often deliberately frightening ways. Choosing appropriate images that don't needlessly add to your fear will be important. You may want your helper to screen movies ahead of time. Suggested movies include *The Dentist* and *The Secret Lives of Dentists*. Many TV commercials feature dentists and dental work. You could tape a few of these commercials and watch the most anxiety-provoking segments repeatedly. Your dentist may have training videos that show dental work being done that you could borrow. Or, instructional videos may be available from a dental school or a school for dental hygiene if one exists in your area. In addition, there are Web sites that have brief videos of dental work (such as www.iseek.org/sv/13000.jsp?id=100298).

For photos of dental items and situations, search Google's images site (http://images.google.com) using keywords such as "dentist," "dental," "dental treatment," "dental tools," and "dentist drill." There are many Web sites that include photos of dental items. Try www.fotosearch.com/stock-photos/pictures/images/dentistry, for example. You could also look at a library, dental school library, or bookstore for textbooks and journals with a dental theme.

dental tools and instruments

Many dental tools are available in the dental section of a drugstore. You can also look in your yellow pages for dental supply stores or search the Internet for businesses that sell dental supplies and equipment. Finally, your dentist may be able to recommend places where you can purchase dental supplies.

dental settings

Most communities will have a variety of dental settings. These include dentists' offices (and dentists' chairs), dentists' waiting rooms, and possibly a clinic at a dental or dental hygienists' school. Many dental schools have a museum where various dental objects may be displayed. If you let your dentist know about your fear, you could ask if it would be possible to have a visit without getting any work done, just so you could have an opportunity to sit in the dentist's chair and have a look at some of the instruments that dentists use. Dentists may also be able to spread out dental work over a few appointments, allowing you more of an opportunity for gradual exposure. Your dentist and dental hygienist may be happy to go at your pace, explaining things as they go along.

dental sounds

People with a fear of dentists often fear the sounds heard at the dentist's office. Some of our clients with dental fears have found that the sound of an electric toothbrush replicates the sound or experience of a dentist's drill fairly closely. If you plug your ears with earplugs when using an electric toothbrush, the experience may be even more realistic.

There are also Web sites that have sound libraries available to download, including sounds found in a dentist's office. For example, the site http://monkeyfilter.com/link.php/3479 contains realistic dental sounds that can be downloaded for free. Another site, www.audio sparx.com/sa/display/sounds.cfm/sound_group_iid.819/requesttime out.480, contains dental sounds that can be downloaded for a small fee. Alternatively, consider asking your dentist if you could get a tape recording of a dental procedure; or, if a friend is going to the dentist, he or she may be able to get permission from an understanding dentist to make a brief audiotape (or even a videotape) of the experience.

exposure ideas for blood phobias

Exposure practices for blood phobias typically include looking at photos and videos of blood and related triggers, as well as confronting blood-related situations in real life. Here are some ideas for images, items, and settings you might use for your exposures.

blood-related images, photos, and videos

There are a number of TV shows now that show fairly graphic scenes of blood. TLC's *The Operation* is one suggestion. Videotape an episode and find scenes that are particularly anxiety provoking. You can then play back the scenes as many times as you need to. Check out your local video rental store for movies that have scenes with blood. Ask the video store clerk for some suggestions. There is no end to such films. There are also many video games now available that have fairly realistic scenes involving blood that you could consider using as an exposure item. On the Internet, search Google's images site (http://images.google.com) using keywords such as "bloody," "blood," "wound," "surgery," "knife wound," or "cut." Some of these images may be quite distressing to start with, so you may want your helper to screen them ahead of time.

settings for blood-related exposures

There are a number of settings or situations that provide opportunities for exposure to blood. For example, go with a friend when he or she donates blood or has a blood test done. Donate blood yourself. Have blood drawn at a medical lab (this will require a doctor's requisition). As you try to generate ideas, consider exposures to real blood (buy a steak and drain off the blood or prick your finger with a lancet, available in pharmacies) or to theatrical blood (available at joke shops, theatrical stores, costume shops, and Halloween supply stores). These places will often also supply other blood-related items and materials to create fake cuts and wounds. Consider filling a syringe or some other small container with theatrical blood to carry around with you. There are Internet sites that supply recipes for making very realistic-looking fake blood. Here is one such recipe, found at www.shades-of-night.com/painneck/blood.html:

1 tablespoon cocoa powder

½ cup water

3 to 4 tablespoons corn syrup

½ to 1 teaspoon red food coloring

2 drops yellow or green food coloring

Thoroughly mix the cocoa powder into the water. Using warm water may help. Then add the remaining ingredients, blending the mixture well. Skim the bubbles and chocolate "scum" off the top with a tissue. Wiped onto a cloth or article of clothing, this theatrical blood looks very realistic. (It may stain clothing, so be careful.) It splatters like real blood, and when it dries, it even looks like real dried blood.

exposure ideas for injection and needle phobias

Here are some suggestions for where you might find photos and videos involving needles, injections, and blood tests, as well as ideas for confronting these situations directly.

needle and injection images, photos, and videos

Movies with good injection scenes include *Trainspotting, Panic in Needle Park, Dead Man Walking, Philadelphia,* and *Drugstore Cowboy.* Consider renting one of these movies and repeatedly watching only the injection scenes until your anxiety lessens. Your pharmacy or local diabetes clinic may have educational videos available to teach people how to give insulin injections. These videos will have images of needles and injections. There are even some videos on this topic available on the Internet. Have a look at the site www.lantus.com/information/injection/index.jsp?id=5030#. Or, a medical library may have instructional videos geared at teaching people how to take blood, how to put in an IV, or how to give an injection. You may also want to consider movies or videos that involve subjects like tattooing, piercing, or acupuncture. On the Internet, search Google's images site (http://images.google.com) using keywords such as "needle," "injection," "IV," "syringe," "immunization," "vaccination," or "acupuncture."

needle- and injection-related situations

Speak to your doctor about your fear of needles and injections. You may be able to receive immunizations for various infections such as hepatitis A or B. Consider getting a flu shot. Your doctor may be able to supply you with a few needles that you could take home and use as exposure items. You can examine them and start to get used to them. You might also be able to obtain needles at your local pharmacy. Go along and watch when your helper or a friend visits the doctor for a vaccination or a flu shot. Or, go along and watch when your helper or a friend has blood taken or gets a piercing. Consider getting acupuncture or watching someone else receive acupuncture. If you know someone who has a condition that requires regular injections (such as insulin for diabetes), ask if you could watch the injection process.

<hr>

exercise: making a list of possible exposures

Now, have a look at the hierarchy you created in chapter 3 and write down a list of the items you'll need for your exposures and where you might be able to find them, using this chapter as a guide. Remember, you don't have to get all of the materials ahead of time. You can get them as you go. You may find that once treatment is under way, some items you initially thought would be helpful become less so. You may also find the opposite is true—as you progress with your exposure exercises, you discover new ideas, situations, or objects that cause fear. You may want to add these to your hierarchy. Because tracking down items, images, and settings for your exposure practice will require you to encounter things and situations that may cause you great distress, you should consider having your helper assist in this process. You should go over your hierarchy and your list of needed items with your helper and discuss who will get what, leaving some of the more anxiety-provoking items for your helper to screen ahead of time. This is why it's important to have a helper who doesn't have the same fear you do.

It's normal to feel anxious as you anticipate confronting your fear. In fact, reading through this chapter may have been a bit of an exposure exercise in itself. For some people, even seeing the word "blood" or "needle" can be frightening. Remember, you can expect to feel anxious as you work on your exposure exercises. Remember, too, that often these exercises can leave you feeling drained, tired, tearful, or irritable. Some people find they feel more tense afterward and have to deal with headaches or muscle stiffness. These are all common reactions on the path to recovery. To help cope with these potential reactions, plan to reward yourself after each exposure exercise. Make a point of going for a walk, getting together with friends, listening to some of your favorite music, or soaking in a warm bath. Consider buying yourself a treat, such as a new outfit or dinner at a great restaurant, to reward yourself for a job well done after tackling a really tough step on your hierarchy. Facing your fear isn't easy. Remember to be kind to yourself along the way.

summary

Before beginning to work your way up the exposure hierarchy you created in chapter 3, it's important to make sure you're well prepared. In this chapter, we discussed the potential benefits of enlisting a helper, who may be a friend, a family member, or a professional therapist. We also reviewed the importance of gathering materials to use in your exposure practices and suggested a number of resources available to that end. Following the guidelines and suggestions in this chapter will help you lay the foundation for successful treatment.

5

confronting your fear

It's a natural response for people to avoid situations that make them uncomfortable or to take steps to reduce their discomfort in some other way. The drive to be comfortable leads people to take medication for a headache, run cold water over a burn, eat when hungry, sleep when tired, or have a glass of wine when feeling shy at a party. The greater the discomfort, the stronger the urge to take steps to reduce it. Therefore, one of the most noticeable features of any phobia is the tendency to avoid feared situations or to find ways of protecting oneself from feeling overly anxious or frightened in these situations.

why avoidance is a problem

Often, our attempts to feel comfortable are aimed at achieving immediate relief, sometimes at the expense of long-term relief. For example, although many sleep medications are effective for improving sleep on any particular night, discontinuing these medications after a period of regular use is often associated with "rebound" insomnia caused by withdrawal from the medication. In other words, these medications offer a short-term solution to insomnia that may actually increase the problem in the future, when the person stops taking the medication. In the same way, avoiding or escaping from a feared situation leads to immediate relief but makes it more likely that you'll continue to have fear when you encounter the situation in the future.

As we discuss in chapter 7, fear and anxiety are often triggered by negative predictions and assumptions that a situation is dangerous in some way. Examples of such predictions include beliefs that you will faint, that a needle will be painful, that you will be overwhelmed with feelings of fear or disgust, or that a dentist will hurt you. In fact, any prediction of danger or threat can lead to feelings of anxiety or fear. By avoiding a feared situation, you never have a chance to find out whether your prediction is in fact true, whether the outcome is as bad as you expected it to be, and whether you are able to cope with the situation. Just as avoiding dogs almost guarantees that someone won't overcome a fear of dogs, avoiding blood, needles, doctors, or dentists will ensure that your fear is maintained over time. Only through repeated exposure to the situation will you start to experience some long-term relief from your fear.

what to expect during exposure therapy

Can you think of a situation or object that was a source of fear or anxiety in the past but is no longer a problem? For example, were you ever nervous about public speaking or starting a new job? How about skiing, swimming, or riding a bicycle for the first time? If you can't think of a fear you overcame, try to think of a fear that someone close to you overcame in the past. How did you (or the other person) manage to overcome the fear? Chances are that the fear was overcome through confronting the situation until it became easier.

Though exposure is one of the most powerful ways to overcome almost any fear, the process isn't easy. Exposure practices can be uncomfortable, time-consuming, and tiring. If you have a history of passing out upon exposure to blood, injections, and related situations, there is a risk of fainting during your exposure practices. (We'll return to this issue shortly. Also, chapter 6 is devoted to the topic of preventing fainting during exposure practices.) As mentioned in chapter 4, practicing exposures may make you feel anxious, tired, or irritable.

However, it's not all bad news. Many people have a great sense of satisfaction and even excitement following each practice, especially when they start to notice their fear decreasing as a result of exposure. A sense of freedom may also emerge as you begin to realize that situations that were previously off-limits are now a possibility. For most people, the temporary increase in discomfort is manageable, and it's almost always well worth it.

Starting a program of exposure is a lot like starting a new exercise program. When you first begin exercising, the results are not always pleasant. You may feel sore after working out, and you may initially feel more tired. It's only after a few weeks of regular exercise that you start to notice the benefits, including more energy, increased strength, weight loss, and a decreased risk of various illnesses. The same is true for exposure. If you can tolerate some initial discomfort, you'll quickly start to see the benefits—including a reduction in fear and anxiety and an increase in the range of things that you can do comfortably.

dealing with fainting or feelings of faintness

As discussed in chapter 1, phobias of blood, needles, and related situations are the only phobias that are often associated with fainting. In fact, more than half the people who have these phobias have a history of fainting in the feared situation. Many others report having come close to fainting in the past.

If you have no history of fainting or feeling faint, the strategies in this chapter can be used as they are described. However, if you do have a history of fainting, we have a few additional recommendations:

Make sure you read chapter 6 before trying the exposure practices described in this chapter. Although exposure alone is an effective treatment for fears of blood, needles, doctors, and dentists, combining the exposure strategies with the muscle tension exercises described in chapter 6 will help to prevent fainting during your practices. Preventing fainting will make the whole process easier.

Check with your doctor to make sure that it's safe for you to faint. For most people, fainting on occasion in a controlled situation is perfectly safe. However, if you have certain medical conditions (for example, cardiac disease), fainting may be risky. If you have a history of fainting, we recommend clearing this treatment with your family doctor before beginning your exposure practices.

Take precautions to protect yourself in case you faint. The biggest risk in fainting is the possibility of injuring yourself. If you have a history of fainting, all exposures should be done with someone else in the room, particularly early in your treatment when the risk of fainting is still an issue. Make sure you're sitting down so you don't fall down. If you do fall over and are on your back, your helper should roll you onto your side (just in case you vomit).

getting the most out of exposure

At this point, it would be perfectly natural for you to be skeptical about whether exposure can work for you. Chances are that your previous experiences with exposure to your feared situations have been negative—filled with anxiety, fear, embarrassment, and perhaps fainting. Fortunately, there are important differences between the types of exposure experiences you may have had in the past and the ways in which exposure is carried out in therapy. This section provides a number of guidelines for ensuring that exposure works for you.

plan practices in advance

It's useful to decide in advance when and where you're going to practice and what you'll do during your practices. Schedule your exposure practices on your calendar, just as you would an appointment. That way, you'll be more likely to follow through with the plan. Make sure your helper is available as well. If your practices require you to have contact with your doctor or dentist, you'll need to arrange that in advance. If you're practicing at home, make sure that potential distractions are eliminated. For example, if you have young children, schedule your practices when they are away, asleep, or otherwise occupied.

take steps at a pace that works for you

Each person must decide how quickly to move through the steps on his or her hierarchy. Practicing easier items for longer (and taking steps more gradually) has some advantages: The anxiety and fear you experience during your practices will probably be more manageable. You'll also be less likely to panic or faint. However, there are also disadvantages to going slowly: The slower you take steps, the longer it will take you to overcome your fear. And because you'll notice changes more slowly, you may start to lose motivation to push yourself.

Again, the analogy of physical exercise is useful. If you push yourself to work out more strenuously, you'll see bigger changes in your fitness level, and the changes will occur more quickly. If you lift lighter weights and spend less time on the treadmill, you'll still notice changes, but they'll take longer and be more modest.

Our recommendation is to take steps as quickly as you are willing to. However, if you prefer to take things more slowly, that's fine. As mentioned in chapter 1, many people with blood and needle phobias are able to overcome their fears with just a few hours of exposure. If you push yourself to practice the items on your hierarchy more quickly, or to practice items that are more difficult, you'll see changes more quickly. The worst thing that may happen is that you'll feel more anxiety and fear (and if you have a history of fainting, you may also increase the likelihood of fainting). If an item is too difficult, you can always change the practice to something easier. There's no danger in taking steps quickly, other than the possibility of feeling more uncomfortable.

minimize surprises

Exposure works best when the practices are predict-able. For example, if you were afraid of snakes and some-one surprised you by throwing a snake at you, that kind of exposure wouldn't work! On the other hand, if you were told that there was a harmless snake in a nearby room and you had the opportunity to approach it gradu-ally, at your own pace and with no surprises, your fear would slowly decrease.

The same is true when dealing with fears of blood, needles, doctors, and dentists. It's best to know as much about the situation as possible. For example, before start-ing an exposure practice with a dentist, it's good to know how long the appointment will take, what's going to hap-pen, and what each procedure is likely to feel like. Mak-ing the exposure predictable is especially important early in your treatment. You can always test yourself later with some less predictable exposures, such as having a dental appointment and not asking any questions at the start.

longer exposures are better than shorter exposures

The most effective exposures are ones that last long enough for your fear to come down to no more than a mild or moderate level. Ideally, you should try to stay in the sit-uation until your fear has decreased. That may take a few minutes, or it may take an hour or more. The problem with brief exposures is that they can sometimes strengthen a person's fear by reinforcing the belief, "When I'm in the situation I feel terrible, and when I leave I feel much better." By staying in the situation until your fear has decreased, you'll learn that you can eventually be in the situation and not experience significant fear.

For some practices, it may be difficult to prolong the exposure. For example, if you're fearful of getting an injection, it's difficult to stretch the experience beyond a minute or two. However, it will be easy to extend the length of the exposure for other practices. Here are some ways to extend your exposure practices:

- ◊ Watch a video of an injection over and over again until your feelings of anxiety, disgust, and faintness have subsided.

- ◊ Schedule a full physical with your family doctor, rather than just a quick appointment.

- ◊ Have your dental work done at a dental school's training clinic, where appointments tend to take longer (students take longer to clean patients' teeth and may have to have their work checked by their instructor, which may also slow things down).

- ◊ Schedule two dental appointments back-to-back, just to get the practice (but note that your dental insurance may not pay for this).

- ◊ Practice looking at blood for an extended period.

- ◊ If you're getting a blood test, see if the nurse or doctor will take a bit longer on each step in the process and perhaps take some blood from each arm, instead of just one arm. (Of course, a practice this difficult may not be possible until later in your treatment.)

◊ For fear of having your blood pressure taken, practice having blood pressure tests over and over for as long as it takes for your anxiety to decrease.

schedule your practices close together

Exposure works best when practices are scheduled close together. We are not simply suggesting that spacing exposures closer together leads to faster improvements (though it does). What we're suggesting is that spacing exposures close together actually leads to better outcomes. For example, exposures scheduled once per day for five days will work better than exposures scheduled once per week over five weeks.

It may be difficult to get an injection every day, but most other types of exposure are easier to schedule on a more regular basis. If exposures are too spread out, each practice will be like starting over; however, exposure practices scheduled close together build on one another. Ideally, you should try to practice at least several times per week until your fear has decreased. For example, if you're fearful of getting a physical, you'll see more improvement if you schedule three or four physicals in a single week than if you have a physical every couple of weeks over a period of a few months. Here are some suggestions for how you can schedule your exposures closely together:

- ◇ Schedule dentist appointments (for example, for a checkup) three times per week for a two-week period.

- ◇ Look at a videotape of injections for an hour each evening until it no longer makes you feel anxious or faint.

- ◇ Visit a friend in the hospital twice per day over the next week.

- ◇ Visit a blood donor clinic four times over the next week.

- ◇ Use a finger prick blood test kit to take a bit of blood from several fingers every day over the next two weeks.

eliminate safety behaviors

People with phobias often engage in various behaviors designed to protect them from feeling anxious in the situations they fear. Here are some examples of such safety behaviors:

- ◇ Looking away while getting an injection

- ◇ Offering to get your friend something from the cafeteria while visiting him or her in the hospital (with the true purpose of leaving the hospital room due to fear)

◊   Withholding information from your doctor to minimize the chances of having to get certain tests

◊   Listening to music during dental treatment

◊   Lying to your dentist about pain in a tooth to avoid having to get a filling

◊   Insisting on lying down when blood is drawn

◊   Always attending doctor or dentist appointments with a friend or family member

Most people use simple safety behaviors to help manage their anxiety, and often such behaviors are not a problem. For example, for most people, there's often nothing wrong with looking away during a blood test. However, if your fear is extreme and it interferes with your life, it's much better to gradually reduce your reliance on these safety behaviors. In the short term they help you feel comfortable, but in the long term they help feed your belief that the situation is threatening or dangerous. We recommend that you gradually reduce your reliance on these behaviors as you work through the items on your hierarchy (particularly later in your treatment).

practice in different situations and with different triggers

Exposure seems to work best when practices occur in a variety of settings and with a variety of feared objects. For example, if you fear dentists, it's best to schedule appointments with more than one dentist, or for more than one procedure. Otherwise, you may find that you experience a reduction of fear for only that one dentist or procedure. In addition to scheduling dentist appointments, you can also make a point of watching videos showing dental treatment and role-play simple dental procedures with your helper. (For example, have your helper look at your teeth with a dental mirror while you lie back in a reclining chair.) Here are some other examples of how you can vary the situations and triggers used for exposure practices:

- ◆ Visit your doctor for a number of different procedures, such as blood tests, physicals, removal of a wart, and having your blood pressure tested.

- ◆ Schedule physicals with a number of different doctors.

- ◆ Look at blood in several different formats, including in bags at a blood bank, in tubes at a blood lab, on a bleeding finger at home, on video, and so on.

- ◆ Get blood tests from a number of different nurses in several different labs.

- ◆ Schedule dental cleanings or other procedures with several different dentists and hygienists.

don't fight your fear

Rather than fighting your fear or making a conscious effort to force your symptoms to go away, try to
just let your fear symptoms come and go. The more effort
you put into fighting your fear, the longer you'll keep it
there. If you experience uncomfortable symptoms, such as
faintness, a racing heart, or sweating, just let them pass
without actively fighting them. Notice the symptoms and
then turn your attention back to what's going on.

how to know when treatment is finished

Your treatment will be finished when you can comfortably expose yourself to the situations you currently
fear. As long as you continue to experience significant
fear, the possibility of your fear worsening again will be
elevated, particularly if you don't have the opportunity to
encounter the feared situation for an extended period of
time. However, note that it's perfectly normal to be nervous before certain types of medical or dental procedures.
Most people would be anxious before undergoing major
surgery, for example. Remember, the goal of treatment is
to reduce your fear to a normal level so that it no longer
interferes with your life; the goal is not to eliminate all
fear of medical or dental situations.

exposure case examples

In this section, we describe the use of exposure to treat
phobias of needles, blood, dentists, and doctors. Each case

example describes the specific treatment program that was used, which should make it easier for you to develop a program for overcoming your fear, based on your own hierarchy.

Roxy—needles, injections, and blood tests

Roxy's fear of needles began when she was about ten years old. Before that, she was able to get injections and blood tests comfortably. She could remember very clearly the day her fear began. She was with her mother, visiting her family doctor for a routine physical. When it came time to have blood taken, her mother mentioned to Roxy that she could look away if she wanted to. Although her mother's intention was to comfort Roxy, her comment had the opposite effect. Roxy thought, "Why would I want to look away? Is this something I should be afraid of?" She became very nervous and was relieved when the appointment was finally over.

A few years later, Roxy needed stitches after cutting her hand with a kitchen knife. While getting stitched up, she fainted for the first time. Over the next few years, Roxy fainted several more times during routine blood tests, vaccinations, and other procedures involving needles. Even scenes from movies and television involving injections made her feel faint. Lying down seemed to reduce her faintness, and it usually prevented her from losing consciousness as well.

Through her twenties, Roxy was able to successfully avoid needles most of the time. She rarely saw her family doctor for fear of needing a blood test. At the dentist's, she insisted on having all dental work done without an anesthetic. Fortunately, her health was good, and there was little need for her to confront needles.

However, by the time she turned thirty, Roxy was beginning to think it was time to overcome her fear. She and her husband had recently decided to have a baby, and she was terrified to have the blood work she would need during pregnancy. Also, she was considering taking a new job that required her to receive several vaccinations and a full physical exam, including blood work. Her fear was beginning to interfere with her life, and it was time to do something about it.

At her first therapy session, Roxy's therapist conducted a thorough assessment and worked with Roxy to develop an exposure hierarchy. Given her history of fainting, Roxy and her therapist decided that exposure with applied muscle tension (to prevent fainting) would be the most appropriate treatment for her fear (see chapter 6 for a full description of applied muscle tension procedures). In that first session, Roxy was taught how to tense all the muscles in her body to raise her blood pressure. During the first week, she practiced the exercises for about five or ten minutes at a time several times per day, at home and in her office at work. Over the course of the week, the exercises became easier.

At her next treatment session, Roxy and her therapist introduced exposure practices. Before each practice,

Roxy used the applied tension exercises, and she continued to use them during the exposure practices, particularly when she noticed feelings of faintness. That session focused on exposure to photos of people getting injections, as well as watching a videotape of someone having blood drawn. Roxy watched the video repeatedly for about an hour. During the first thirty minutes she felt quite faint, but the feeling subsided by the end of the hour, until she was able to watch it with minimal anxiety or faintness.

Over the next week, Roxy practiced watching the video at home for about an hour each day. For the first few days, she included the applied tension exercises to minimize any feelings of faintness that might occur. After that, she decided to watch the video without using the tension exercises. She was relieved to discover that she no longer needed to tense her muscles. Feelings of faintness were no longer a problem for this particular practice.

Roxy was ready to move on to the next step. At her next therapy session, her therapist had everything needed to expose Roxy to the types of things she might encounter during an injection or blood test. The session took place in a medical exam room, and the therapist was wearing a lab coat. Roxy repeatedly practiced having her arm tied with a tourniquet, followed each time by her therapist disinfecting the inside of her elbow with an alcohol swab. Next, Roxy practiced holding a sterilized needle to a vein on the inside of her elbow (without breaking the skin). When she was comfortable with this step, she allowed her therapist to hold the needle to her arm. Through the first part of the session, Roxy used the applied tension exercises to combat her faintness, but by the end of the session she was able to do the exposure exercises without applied tension. For homework, Roxy practiced exposure to the tourniquet and alcohol swabs for about thirty minutes each day (with her husband's assistance).

At the next session, it was time to practice exposure to a real blood test. Her therapist was located in a medical office building that had a lab where Roxy could have blood work done. He arranged for her to work with a particular technician who had considerable experience in taking blood from people with needle phobias. Roxy's family doctor agreed to provide several requisitions for blood work. These were necessary for the lab to be able to take the blood. Roxy's therapist was present at the first visit to the lab. Roxy practiced her applied tension exercises for about ten minutes before meeting with the lab technician. During her blood test, she continued to tense her muscles, while being careful to leave her "needle arm" relaxed. She was thrilled that she was able to have blood taken from both arms without fainting.

For homework, she returned with her husband to the lab twice more for additional blood tests, each time with a different technician. During the second visit, Roxy was able to have her blood drawn without using the tension exercises. She met one more time with her therapist to discuss her progress. She was now much more comfortable with the idea of having blood work done during her pregnancy, and she had scheduled the vaccinations and physical for her new job. Roxy had conquered her fear of needles in less than a month.

Zack—blood

Zack's fear of blood began when he fainted while watching a surgery film during a high school biology class. He had always felt a bit queasy around blood, but his fear had been manageable until the time he fainted. Zack started to avoid a number of situations such as having blood drawn, watching medical shows on television, visiting hospitals, talking about medical procedures, and handling raw meat. Although he rarely had to encounter these situations, his life was about to change. He had recently been accepted into medical school and was deciding whether to accept the offer or turn it down because of his fear. Zack decided to get treatment for his blood phobia. If he could overcome his fear before school started (about three months from the time he started treatment), he would accept the offer to study medicine.

Zack's first session began with an assessment, after which an exposure hierarchy was developed. Items near the top of his hierarchy included having blood drawn, seeing someone else bleeding, and watching surgery (live or on video). Moderately difficult items included watching others have blood drawn, holding tubes of blood, and looking at bags of blood. Easier items included looking at tubes of blood from a distance and cutting up raw beef for a stir-fry. Because of Zack's history of fainting, his therapist recommended including the applied tension exercises (described in chapter 6). Zack and his therapist spent a few minutes at the end of the session reviewing instructions for the applied tension procedures. Over the next week, Zack practiced the applied tension exercises daily.

The following week, Zack and his therapist had scheduled a two-hour exposure session. Because Zack was willing to start with some of the more difficult items on his hierarchy, they skipped some of the easier practices. The session began with Zack watching as his therapist used a finger prick blood test kit (the type that someone with diabetes might use to check blood sugar) to draw blood from her own finger. Initially, Zack was able to use the applied tension exercises to control his feelings of faintness. However, after about a minute, he started to feel light-headed and sweaty. A few seconds later, he fainted. Zack was unconscious for about thirty seconds. When he regained consciousness, he was quite woozy and disoriented. He and his therapist decided to end the session a half hour early. Although Zack was unwilling to practice any exposure homework over the next week, he agreed to continue practicing the tension exercises.

The day before his next appointment, Zack called to cancel. He was discouraged about what had happened at the last session and was thinking about discontinuing his treatment. His therapist encouraged Zack to keep his appointment, offering reassurance that Zack would not be forced to do anything before he was ready. Zack agreed to come in for another two-hour exposure session.

At the next session, his therapist suggested that they begin with some easier items from Zack's hierarchy.

They spent the first half hour looking at and then holding a tube of blood. Zack's anxiety gradually decreased, and his feelings of faintness were mild. He was then ready to once again watch his therapist prick her finger while he used the tension exercises. This time, he didn't faint. His therapist then pricked several more fingertips and encouraged Zack to watch the blood on her fingers. Although his anxiety level was quite high, he was successfully able to prevent himself from fainting. Over the course of the next half hour, Zack's anxiety decreased significantly. In the remaining hour of the session, Zack practiced pricking his own finger and then practiced letting his therapist prick his finger. At one point he felt as though he might faint, but the feeling passed after he lay down for a few minutes. Once the faintness passed, he resumed the exposure exercises until his anxiety decreased. For homework over the coming week, Zack practiced the finger prick tests daily with the help of his parents and his girlfriend.

The following week, Zack and his therapist practiced watching several surgery videos, at first using the applied tension exercises, and later watching them without tensing. At the end of the two hours, Zack was able to watch videos depicting cardiac surgery, removal of a facial mole, and a patient receiving stitches, all with only minimal anxiety.

In the end, Zack was quite happy with his progress, and he was glad he had stuck with the treatment. He decided that he would attend medical school after all. Although he was still nervous about watching live surgery, he decided to work on that fear on his own, after starting medical school. His therapy ended after only three sessions.

Jacob—dentists

Jacob had been fearful of the dentist for as long as he could remember. As a child, his parents forced him to go to the dentist once a year. As soon as he became an adult, he stopped going on a regular basis and only saw a dentist if he had a problem that was causing him pain (which happened about every five years). When he did see the dentist, he insisted on being knocked out with a general anesthetic. His main concern was that the experience would be painful; he remembered having a number of uncomfortable visits to the dentist as a child.

By the time Jacob decided to seek treatment at age forty, he had several cavities that needed to be filled and his teeth hadn't been cleaned for years. His children were aware of his fear, and he worried that some of his fear might rub off on them. He decided to confront his fear on his own.

Jacob began by finding a dentist who specialized in treating anxious patients. He was able to get a referral from his wife's dentist. When he made the appointment, he had a choice of several hygienists, so he requested to see the one with the reputation for being the most gentle. At his appointment, he was told that he would likely need several more visits. He had several teeth to fill and one that was likely to require a root canal and crown.

Also, because his teeth hadn't been cleaned in many years, it would likely take a few appointments just to get his teeth cleaned.

When he made his first appointment, Jacob asked whether the dentist and hygienist could begin with less frightening procedures, such as examining his teeth and taking X-rays, and save more difficult procedures such as cleanings, injections, and fillings for subsequent appointments. In fact, the dentist offered to spend an entire appointment just helping Jacob get used to the feeling of having various dental instruments (mirror, probe, scaler, suction tube, and so forth) in his mouth.

Jacob used several strategies to manage his fear. First, he decided to focus just on the procedures he would have done at each appointment, rather than thinking about all the dental work he needed to have done. He also thought about how his wife, coworkers, and friends often told him that the discomfort they experience at the dentist is always manageable, and how the procedures used during dental treatment have changed since he was younger. Finally, he asked the dentist and hygienist to describe to him what procedures would be done, what they were likely to feel like, and how long they would take.

Jacob had a total of six visits to the dentist over a three-week period. Although the first visit was frightening, he was reassured because he knew he wouldn't have any dental work done that day. With each visit, his anxiety improved. After having his teeth cleaned and his cavities filled, he decided to get his root canal and crown done. Although terrified of the procedure, he was reassured when his dentist said that the discomfort would be no worse than that he experienced during the other procedures. In the end, he felt almost no pain despite the reputation root canals have for being painful. He figured that if he could survive a root canal, he could handle anything. He scheduled a checkup for six months later.

Ella—doctors and hospitals

Ella had been afraid of visiting doctors and hospitals since she was a teenager, though she was unsure what initially triggered the fear. There were a number of reasons she avoided seeing doctors. She was uncomfortable being examined and undergoing tests and, to some extent, was afraid she might find out she had a problem that she didn't know she had. She wasn't sure why she didn't like hospitals, but she avoided them at all costs, even if it meant not visiting friends and relatives in the hospital. Now, at age fifty-five, Ella had become increasingly concerned about her phobia. She was at an age when it seemed more important than ever to have regular medical checkups. Also, her parents were older, and she worried that they might soon need to spend time in a hospital and that she wouldn't be able to visit them. She finally decided to seek treatment when her husband was scheduled to have his hip replaced.

Ella's treatment began with developing two hierarchies—one for doctor visits and the other for hospitals. The doctor hierarchy included a list of items varying in difficulty. The hierarchy took into account the variables

that contributed to her fear, including the sex of the doctor (female doctors were easier than males), the age of
the doctor (doctors younger than forty and older than
sixty made her more anxious), the type of procedure
being done (she was most nervous about procedures used
to detect cancer, such as a mammogram), and the type of
doctor (family doctors were easier than specialists). The
hospital hierarchy included items ranging in difficulty
from relatively easy (for example, spending time in the
lobby or cafeteria of a hospital) to more difficult (for
example, walking through the halls in the emergency
room or visiting someone in a hospital room).

Ella decided to start with her fear of doctors. She
made appointments for physical exams three times per
week over a two-week period. The first two exams were
with her family doctor, who was aware of Ella's fear. The
next four exams were with other doctors (recommended
by her family doctor), starting with female physicians and
working up to male physicians. Ella also arranged to have
a number of tests done, including blood work, a
mammogram, and a colonoscopy. Over the course of
these two weeks, her fear of doctors decreased to a moderate level. Ella decided to continue her exposure practices with doctors about once per week over the next
month while also starting to confront her fear of
hospitals.

During the next few weeks, Ella made a point of visiting hospitals about four times per week for an hour or
two, usually on her way home from work. She visited the
hospital where her husband was scheduled to have his

surgery, as well as several others. She began with the easier items on her hierarchy (for example, visiting her family doctor, who was a woman in her early fifties) and
worked her way up to the more difficult items (for example, seeing a young male dermatology resident for a spe-
cialist appointment). Eventually, she had practiced all of
the items on her hierarchy except for visiting a loved one
in the hospital; at the time, she had no friends or relatives who were hospital patients. However, when her husband had his surgery, she was able to visit him daily with
only minimal anxiety.

exercise: exposure to
your feared situations

Of all the exercises described in this book, this one is the
most important. Completing this exercise will ultimately
lead to a reduction in your fear. This exercise is also
among the most difficult in the book. It requires time and
patience, as well as a willingness to feel uncomfortable, at
least temporarily. Unlike some of the other exercises in
this book, this is not an exercise you can complete in a few
minutes. Instead, you'll need to practice for several hours
over the course of a few days or a few weeks to complete
this exercise. If you have a history of fainting upon
encountering blood, needles, or related situations, don't
complete this exercise until you have read chapter 6. For
those who faint or even just feel faint, we recommend only

completing this exercise in conjunction with the applied tension techniques described in chapter 6.

Essentially, this exercise involves exposing yourself to the situations on your hierarchy, using the strategies described in this chapter along with those in chapters 3 and 4. Remember, your exposures should be planned, structured, predictable, frequent (at least several times per week), and prolonged (ideally lasting until your fear has decreased to a mild or moderate level). The case examples in this chapter illustrate how you might organize your own exposure practices.

Each time you complete an exposure practice, record in your journal how anxious you were before beginning the practice, your anxiety level every five or ten minutes during the practice, and your anxiety level at the end. Use a scale ranging from 0 (no anxiety) to 100 (maximum anxiety). In addition, record what practice you completed (for example, "watching a cardiac surgery video for thirty minutes"), how long it took for your discomfort to decrease, and any other relevant details (for example, whether you fainted during the practice).

troubleshooting

Generally, exposure to feared situations is the most effective way to overcome phobias of blood, needles, and dental and medical situations. However, there are a number of obstacles that can occasionally get in the way. Here are some strategies for dealing with four of the most common obstacles.

finding time to practice

Exposure takes time—a rare commodity for many of us. You may be busy with work, school, raising children, or any number of other activities, making it difficult to find an hour or two to devote to exposure on a given day. If so, we recommend that you schedule your exposure practices just as you would any other activity or appointment in your day. If you have young children, it may be necessary to hire a babysitter. If it's too difficult to practice during the week, increase the amount of practice you do on the weekend. Or, take a vacation day from work to practice. Fortunately, exposure-based treatments tend to work quickly for phobias of blood, needles, doctors, and dentists. Following a few hours of exposure, you will likely notice a reduction in your fear.

your fear is too strong

If your fear is overwhelming during a particular exposure practice, try something a bit easier. If you can't complete a specific exercise, ask yourself, "How can I change this exercise to make it more manageable?" It's better to do an easier practice than to avoid practicing altogether.

small veins that make it difficult to take blood

Some people who fear having blood drawn have good reason for their fear. Specifically, some people have small veins that are hard to find, making it difficult to take blood. As a result, nurses, doctors, and others often try unsuccessfully to take blood from various locations and may end up causing considerable pain and bruising with each attempt. If you have small veins, you should take steps to minimize the "trauma" that normally occurs when you have blood taken. First, make sure that the person drawing your blood is experienced in drawing blood from people with small veins. Second, let the person know that it's generally very difficult to draw your blood from the usual places. If there's another location that tends to work better (for example, your hand), suggest that the person drawing your blood try that location first.

fear that won't come down

There are a number of reasons why your fear may not decrease during a particular practice. First, the practice may not be long enough. Fear reduction can take anywhere from a few minutes to a few hours. If your fear is staying high, make sure you have given it an adequate opportunity to come down. Another factor that may prevent your fear from decreasing is significant life stress (for example, a hectic work schedule, frequent marital conflict, or parenting pressures). If you've had a stressful day and your fear doesn't decrease during practice, try again another day. Finally, it's best not to engage in safety behaviors or subtle avoidance behaviors, such as distraction, during your exposures. These behaviors may keep your anxiety higher over the course of your exposure practice.

summary

Exposure is the treatment of choice for phobias of blood, needles, doctors, and dentists. It works best when practices are prolonged, frequent, predictable, and planned. For people who faint, exposure should be combined with applied muscle tension exercises, which are described in chapter 6. This chapter included four case examples to illustrate how exposure therapy plays out in real life, and we also presented strategies for dealing with some of the most common obstacles that may arise during treatment.

6

preventing fainting

People with blood and needle phobias often faint during exposure to a feared situation. As mentioned earlier, a little more than 50 percent of people with needle phobias have a history of fainting during injections and almost 70 percent of people with blood phobias report fainting upon exposure to blood (Öst 1992). The tendency of these phobias to be associated with fainting is unique; it is very unusual for people with other types of phobias (for example, fears of heights, animals, or flying) to report fainting in the feared situation.

If you tend to faint in your feared situations, practicing exposures can be especially challenging. This chapter will explain exactly what causes fear-induced fainting. We'll also teach you a proven technique to help reduce the possibility of fainting. If fainting isn't a problem for you, you can skip this chapter if you want.

what happens when we faint?

There are two main organ systems in the body that are involved in fainting. One is the cardiovascular system, which includes the heart and blood vessels, and the other is the nervous system, which includes the brain, the spinal cord, and all of the nerves that control the muscles and organs.

the cardiovascular system's role in fainting

In order to stay alert and awake, the brain needs to have a constant flow of oxygen-rich blood. Because the brain is above the heart when we are standing upright, gravity tends to pull blood away from the brain. Therefore, your blood needs to be under enough pressure to get it up to your brain and to keep it from pooling in your legs, in the same way that water in a two-story house needs to be under pressure to get a good flow in the upstairs shower. That blood pressure is maintained by the muscles in the walls of your blood vessels and by the rate and power with which your heart beats.

When the muscles in the walls of your blood vessels contract, they narrow the diameter of the blood vessels, causing an increase in your blood pressure. If that muscles become relaxed, blood vessels increase in diameter, resulting in a drop in blood pressure. Blood pressure is also affected by the rate at which your heart beats. If your heart rate slows down, your blood pressure decreases. If your heart rate speeds up, your blood pressure increases.

So relaxed blood vessels and a slow heart rate both result in reduced blood pressure. Reduced blood pressure, in turn, results in pooling of blood in the legs (because that's where gravity pulls it). Pooling of blood in the legs means less blood is available to get to the brain, and that means the brain is deprived of oxygen. A brain without oxygen can't stay alert and can't hold up the body it controls, so fainting occurs.

the nervous system's role in fainting

The nervous system includes all of the nerves to all the organs and muscles in your body. Your nervous system tells your heart how fast to beat and tells the muscles in the walls of your blood vessels how relaxed to be. The specific nerve involved in fear-related fainting is called the *vagus nerve*.

When the vagus nerve is activated, it tells the heart to beat more slowly and tells the muscles of the blood vessel walls to relax. Remember, a slow heart rate and relaxed blood vessel wall muscles result in decreased blood pressure, which ultimately leads to fainting. However, the key thing to remember is that activation of the vagus nerve can result in fainting.

how does a fear of medical situations lead to fainting?

Now you understand the mechanics of fainting, but we still haven't answered the question as to why people faint when they see blood, get an injection, or are overcome with fear at the doctor's office or in the dentist's chair. Although the exact mechanisms are not yet fully understood, we do know that strong emotional reactions such as fear and anxiety (and even extreme sorrow), as well as the threat of physical pain or injury, will activate the vagus nerve. The sight of blood, the thought of a needle, the sound of a dentist's drill, or the smell of a doctor's office can all produce an emotional response strong enough to activate the vagus nerve. Activation of the vagus nerve is much stronger in some people than in others (probably for genetic reasons; Page and Martin 1998), so they are more likely to faint when exposed to emotionally charged objects or situations.

However, fainting in the presence of blood and related situations doesn't require the presence of fear. In a survey of college students, Kleinknecht and Lenz (1989) found that among those who reported a history of fainting upon seeing blood, 38 percent had a full-blown blood phobia, 28 percent were somewhat fearful of blood (but didn't have a full phobia), and 34 percent reported no fear of blood. In other words, some people occasionally faint when they see blood, despite reporting not being afraid of blood.

how can fainting be a good thing?

You may be wondering why humans would develop a tendency to faint in the presence of blood and injury. Although we don't really know the answer, a number of theories exist. One possibility is that, evolutionarily speaking, when our ancestors were living in caves and hunting wild animals to survive, if they became injured and began to bleed, then a drop in blood pressure might actually be good. Blood that is under reduced pressure has less force behind it and therefore flows more slowly and may clot more quickly. So a drop in blood pressure at the sight of one's own blood may have resulted in fainting, but at the same time, it could have kept some of our ancestors from bleeding to death while out on the hunting grounds.

Another possible explanation lies in the fact that wild animals are generally less likely to attack an unconscious victim. Therefore, if our ancestors were attacked by a wild animal and blood was drawn, fainting at the sight of one's own blood may have kept the wild animal from finishing what it started, in turn allowing the victim to survive.

A third possibility is that vasovagal fainting may have developed to promote the development of fear toward certain things. Fainting is an unpleasant experience, and in general, people try to avoid unpleasant experiences and the things that cause them. If things like pain, blood, knives, the teeth of wild animals, and other dangerous threats became associated with fainting, people may have been more likely to develop a fear of these things and in turn would have learned to avoid such situations, resulting in improved survival in the wild.

how does all this apply to my fainting?

While fainting may be helpful at certain dangerous times, it isn't helpful in the situations where you tend to faint. There is no life-threatening danger from watching a bloody scene in a movie, getting an injection or having blood drawn, getting a filling, or having your doctor examine you. Fainting at these times is unhelpful and annoying, to say the least. Learning to prevent fainting at these times would be beneficial.

is it possible to prevent fainting?

How can you learn to control your fainting? Well, it would be great if you could somehow consciously override your vagus nerve and contract the tiny muscles inside the walls of your blood vessels on command to increase blood pressure and in turn prevent blood from pooling in your legs. Unfortunately, you have no direct control over the muscles in the walls of your blood vessels. But you do have control over other muscles in your body—the larger muscles that help move your arms, hands, legs, feet, torso, and neck. These are called *skeletal muscles*.

In the 1980s, psychologist Michael Kozak published two case studies suggesting that tensing the skeletal muscles of the body could prevent fainting in people who fear blood and injury (Kozak and Miller 1985; Kozak and

Montgomery 1981). Following these studies, the Swedish scientist Lars-Göran Öst and his colleagues further developed and tested this method in a number of larger studies (Hellström, Fellenius, and Öst 1996; Öst, Fellenius, and Sterner 1991; Öst and Sterner 1987; Öst, Sterner, and Fellenius 1989). They discovered that tensing these large skeletal muscles can apply enough external force to your blood vessel walls to increase blood pressure sufficiently to prevent fainting. This method of preventing fainting is called *applied tension*, and you can easily learn to do it. As discussed in chapter 5, those people prone to fainting in feared situations should generally use these exercises in conjunction with exposure practices, especially at first.

learning applied tension

Mastering the applied tension method of preventing vasovagal fainting takes practice and may take some time, so be patient. It's often helpful to perfect the technique in a nonfearful setting first. Here's a step-by-step guide to mastering the applied tension technique. Read through all the steps first, then do the practice exercise that follows.

Step 1: Find a quiet and comfortable place in your home where you can be alone without any fear of distraction or intrusion by others. Sit in a comfortable chair or recline on the couch or a bed. Focus on the muscles in your legs, arms, and torso. Now tense those muscles. Make them contract. Hold that contraction until you feel a warm feeling or a "rush" in your head (usually about ten to fifteen seconds), and then relax and rest for about thirty seconds. Repeat the same procedure four more times.

Step 2: Repeat step 1 five times per day, for a total of twenty-five tensing episodes per day. Do this every day for a week. This may seem like a lot of practice, but the better you can get at this technique, the easier it will be when it comes time to put it to work in the real world. You want to practice enough that it becomes automatic. That being said, some people can overdo it. The development of headaches could mean that you're tensing too hard. If this happens, cut back on the intensity of your muscle contractions or reduce the number of tensing episodes you do in a day.

Step 3: Once you've practiced the applied tension exercise for a week in the comfort of your home, you'll be ready to practice it during your exposure exercises. When you're doing an exposure exercise that you know may lead to fainting, look for early warning signs of an oncoming faint (see below) and put your applied tension to work. If one of your exposure exercises involves giving blood, you'll have to learn to relax the arm from which blood is being drawn while tensing all of the other muscles in your body. Practice doing this when you're not having blood drawn first, until you have it perfected.

Step 4: As you work your way up your exposure hierarchy, you'll notice that your anxiety begins to diminish. Remember that strong emotions like anxiety and fear in the presence of blood and related situations turn on the vagus nerve, so as the emotional reaction to your feared object or situation becomes less intense, the tendency for your vagus nerve to become highly activated will diminish. In turn, your tendency to faint will diminish even in the absence of applied tension. As you notice your anxiety diminishing in various exposures, you may want to try the exposures without the applied tension exercises. You may find that the reduced fear response alone is enough to keep you from fainting and that you no longer need to use the applied tension technique. However, you now have the technique memorized and ready to use should you ever need it.

---

exercise: practicing applied tension

Now that you've read the instructions for applied tension, find a quiet spot in your home and begin a practice session as described in step 1, above. Remember, this is a skill that needs to be practiced to be mastered, and just like any other skill, it may take time to perfect it. Once you've completed step 1, move on to steps 2, 3, and 4. In your journal, note each time you practice and record how well the exercise worked for you.

---

identifying warning signs of an impending faint

To use the applied tension technique most effectively, it will be very helpful for you to know when you may be about to faint. There are almost always warning signs in the form of physical symptoms that precede a fainting episode. These symptoms, which will be different for different people, include light-headedness, clamminess, nausea, and hot or cold flushes. It's important for you to pay attention to these early warning signs of an impending fainting episode. Once you can recognize them, you can take action to reverse the fainting process and stop the faint before it happens by using the applied tension techniques described in this chapter.

exercise: identifying early warning signs of fainting

In your journal, make a list of the physical symptoms you feel that tend to warn you of an oncoming fainting episode. Think back to one of your most vivid or most recent fainting (or near-fainting) episodes and recall what physical symptoms you felt that signaled an oncoming faint. Did you get hot and sweaty? Did you get light-headed and dizzy? Did your vision become blurry? Did you feel nauseous? You can use these warning signs to know when to put the applied tension method to work during your exposure exercises, or even during your day-to-day life.

what if I faint during an exposure?

Now that you've reviewed the applied tension method, you know that you can have some control over whether you faint. But there may still be times that, for whatever reason, a fainting episode cannot be prevented. What then? Generally, fainting itself is not dangerous. Most people regain consciousness within seconds. However, falling during a faint can be dangerous, depending on where you are when you faint. As you start to practice your applied tension skills in exposure situations, you should start off by being in fairly safe environments. By that, we mean that you should avoid doing exposures in risky places, like at the top of a flight of stairs, on a balcony, sitting on a high stool, close to sharp or hard objects, or anywhere else where injury would be likely if you do faint.

It's also a good idea to have someone with you, like your helper, in case you faint. If you do faint, your helper should lay you on your side. This is called the *recovery position* and it reduces the risk of harm if you were to vomit while unconscious. A horizontal position will also allow for improved blood flow to your brain, thereby quickening your recovery. Once you feel confident in your ability to recognize the signs of an impending faint soon enough to apply the applied tension technique, you can do exposures in the absence of your helper.

It might also be a wise idea to start off doing your exposures in a more reclined position. This will decrease the blood pressure needed to get blood to your brain, which means that even if your blood pressure does fall with exposure to your feared object or situation, you'll be less likely to faint. And, if you do end up fainting, you won't fall, so you'll be safer. Dental chairs, doctor's examining tables, and blood donation chairs are all made so that the patient can be in a reclined position. As you start your exposures, feel free to ask your doctor, dentist, or lab technician if you can have the work done in a reclined position. As you progress up your exposure hierarchy, consider slowly increasing the incline toward a more vertical position.

can fainting be dangerous?

In very rare cases, fainting can pose a health risk for some people with preexisting medical problems, such as certain heart conditions. If you have any medical concerns about fainting during an exposure, check with your doctor before doing any exposures to be sure that fainting isn't dangerous for you. Also, if you have any concerns that your fainting is not vasovagal (there are many types of fainting), you should discuss this with your doctor to see if any further investigations need to be done with regard to your particular fainting episodes. Some causes of fainting can be serious. Usually, a doctor can tell just by talking to you if yours is a vasovagal faint.

summary

In this chapter you learned what fainting is and how the nervous system and the cardiovascular system interact to cause fainting. By understanding the mechanisms behind fainting, you learned how to lessen your chances of fainting by using applied tension, a technique for increasing blood pressure, thereby reducing pooling of blood in your legs, resulting in sufficient blood flow to your brain. You also learned how to incorporate applied tension into your exposure hierarchy in a safe manner.

7

changing your thoughts

It's not blood, needles, doctors, or dentists that trigger your fear, but rather your perceptions of them. In other words, your interpretations, beliefs, predictions, and associations regarding these situations determine whether you experience fear. Understanding the relationship between perceptions and fear lends some insight into why some people have medical phobias and others don't. Quite simply, people who perceive these situations as threatening or dangerous experience fear, whereas people who perceive them as safe are able to approach such situations with minimal anxiety.

Of course, not all anxious beliefs are untrue. For example, if you have a history of fainting upon exposure to blood, your belief that you're likely to faint the next time you see blood may indeed be a realistic one.

However, many of the beliefs that contribute to phobias are often biased, exaggerated, or unrealistic. For example, although it is true that dental treatment is sometimes uncomfortable, many people overestimate the amount of pain they'll experience next time they go to the dentist. People who fear fainting during a blood test may overestimate just how terrible it would be to actually faint. It is these exaggerated or unrealistic beliefs and assumptions that this chapter is meant to help change.

The strategies described in this chapter are often referred to as *cognitive strategies* or *cognitive therapy*. The word "cognitive" simply refers to processes involving thought, such as ruminating, thinking, imagining, remembering, paying attention, and related processes. Cognitive therapy involves helping people identify their patterns of negative thinking and replace negative thoughts with more balanced or realistic thoughts that are based on a thorough analysis of the evidence concerning the beliefs.

Note that almost all studies on the treatment of blood and needle phobias are based on the exposure strategies discussed in chapter 5 (often combined with the tension exercises described in chapter 6 for those with a history of fainting). Most experts believe that exposure to a feared situation is the most powerful way to combat fear. The techniques described in this chapter are not meant to be used instead of the exposure-based strategies. Rather, they are meant to be used in addition to exposure, or perhaps to give you the courage you need to do the exposure exercises.

Note that the cognitive strategies and exposure may work through similar mechanisms. For example, exposure may well be effective because it provides evidence that challenges anxious beliefs and assumptions. In fact, avoiding feared situations tends to increase the intensity of negative thinking. For example, Kent (1985) found that people with dental anxiety who visit the dentist infrequently are more likely to predict that their next visit to the dentist will be a negative experience, compared to people with the same level of dental anxiety who visit the dentist on a regular basis (probably because they believe they will need more extensive treatment).

The effectiveness of the cognitive strategies described in this chapter is well established for certain types of anxiety problems, including panic disorder, in which people have rushes of panic out of the blue, and social anxiety disorder, in which people experience anxiety in social or performance situations (see Antony and Swinson 2000). However, unlike exposure-based treatments, cognitive therapies have not been studied much for fears of blood, needles, doctors, and dentists. In fact, there have been no large-scale studies on the effectiveness of cognitive therapy on blood and needle phobias in particular, though some initial case studies suggest that these strategies may be useful (Panzarella and Garlipp 1999; Thompson 1999). In the case of dental phobia, however, there are a few larger, well-controlled studies showing that changing your thoughts (often in addition to exposure) can lead to a reduction in dental anxiety (de Jongh et al. 1995; Getka and Glass 1992).

figuring out what you're thinking

One of the most challenging aspects of cognitive therapy is trying to figure out what you are actually thinking. In many cases, the assumptions, perceptions, and predictions that contribute to fear occur very quickly, often outside of our awareness. In fact, the fear we experience in reaction to the situations we fear may seem to occur almost automatically. However, that doesn't mean that our fear is not triggered by our perceptions of the situation.

There are many examples of how our perceptions can influence our behavior even when we're not aware that this is happening. For example, consider the act of driving a car. When you first learn to drive, you need to think carefully about every little thing you do. You must pay attention to what's happening on the road in front of you, but you also need to check your rearview mirror on occasion and attend to what's happening off to the side. You may also check your speedometer, talk to the person in the passenger seat, make sure your feet are on the right pedals, and remember to change gears when necessary. However, over time, driving becomes second nature, and you can do many of these things automatically, paying only minimal attention. That doesn't mean you aren't interpreting your surroundings and making decisions based on your perceptions. It just means that the process is happening automatically. The same is true in the case of phobias. The fear you experience upon exposure to blood, needles, doctors, or dentists may be quick and automatic, but it's probably related to your perception that the situation is dangerous or threatening in some way.

The first step in changing your thoughts is to figure out what they are in the first place. It may be difficult to identify your thoughts at first, but it should become easier with practice. Typically, people with phobias experience anxious thoughts and predictions about the objects and situations they fear. However, they may also experience anxious thoughts about their own anxious reactions (panic attacks, fainting, dizziness, and the like).

thoughts about the feared situation and its effects

Anxious thoughts about a feared object or situation usually involve predictions about what might happen as a direct result of encountering the situation. Here are some examples of such predictions:

- ◊ I'll experience intense pain at the dentist's.

- ◊ I'll find out at the doctor's that I have a serious illness.

- ◊ The doctor or dentist will make a mistake.

- ◊ The anesthesia won't work.

- ◊ I'll get sick from unclean needles or another source of contamination.

- ◊ The treatment I receive may do more harm than good (for example, side effects from medication or mercury from dental fillings).

◊ The doctor, nurse, or dentist will think badly of me for not taking better care of myself.

◊ The doctor will judge me (for example, thinking I'm fat) if I have to expose my body.

thoughts about your anxiety reaction to the feared situation

In addition to fearing the object or situation itself, people with phobias often are fearful of the anxiety symptoms they experience in the presence of their feared situation. For example, people with height phobias often fear getting dizzy in high places, people with a fear of enclosed places often are fearful of experiencing breathlessness in enclosed places, and people with a fear of public speaking often fear experiencing signs of anxiety that might be noticeable to others, such as blushing, sweating, or shaking.

In many cases, people with medical phobias are less frightened of sensations such as blushing, sweating, breathlessness, or a racing heart. However, it's not at all unusual for people with blood or needle fears to be concerned about the possibility of fainting. In one study, 77 percent of people with blood phobia and 48 percent of people with injection phobia reported fearing that they would faint in the situation (Öst 1992). Phobias of blood, needles, doctors, and dentists may also be associated with fear of having a panic attack and not being able to escape, or fear of experiencing overwhelming feelings of disgust.

exercise: identifying your anxious thoughts

In your journal, make a list of the thoughts that you typically have about the situations you fear that involve blood, needles, doctors, or dentists. If you had to encounter your feared situation, what do you fear might happen? What predictions do you make concerning these situations? For each prediction, make a note of how strongly you believe in it. Use a scale ranging from 0 to 100, where 0 means you don't believe the prediction at all and 100 means you completely (or 100 percent) believe the prediction will come true.

strategies for changing anxious thoughts

The goal of cognitive therapy is not simply to replace negative thoughts with positive thoughts, but rather to broaden your thinking, consider all possible outcomes, consider the evidence for your thoughts, and arrive at a more realistic way of viewing the situation. To accomplish this, an initial strategy that can be very useful is simply to stop assuming your beliefs are true. Many people treat their beliefs as though they are facts. Instead, we recommend that you treat your beliefs about blood, needles, doctors, or dentists as guesses about the way things may be. Next, we recommend that you begin to ask yourself questions to help evaluate whether your anxious beliefs are, in fact, true. Ask yourself questions along these lines:

- ◊ Are my beliefs necessarily true?

- ◊ Are there other ways of thinking about this situation?

- ◊ What else might happen, other than what I'm predicting will occur?

- ◊ How might someone who doesn't feel uncomfortable think about this situation?

- ◊ Would my feared outcome really be as bad as I think it would be?

Beginning to question your thoughts is an important step in learning to change them. In the rest of this chapter, we provide additional instructions for learning to think more realistically about the situations you fear.

education

One way of replacing unrealistic thoughts with realistic ones is to ensure you have a sufficient amount of information about your feared situation. For example, if you're convinced that the pain during a dental filling will be unbearable but you can't recall what getting a filling actually feels like, make an effort to learn what you can about the situation. Ask your dentist to explain exactly what the procedure involves and how much discomfort you can expect to feel. Similarly, if you're afraid of experiencing pain during a surgical procedure, find out from your doctor how much discomfort you're likely to actually experience, how long the procedure will last, how you're likely to feel after the procedure is over, what steps you can take to minimize your discomfort, and what you can do to ensure a quick recovery.

Essentially, becoming educated about the situation you fear involves identifying questions that you want answered and then making an attempt to find the answers by talking to your health care professional, talking with others who have had the procedure done, or reading relevant books or articles. The Internet can be a great source of information and statistics, but try to focus on sites that provide balanced information. Try to avoid sites that emphasize only the negative things that may happen. Given your fear, your natural tendency may be to give more weight to negative information you come across than positive information. Beware of that tendency.

exercise: learning about your feared situation

What questions do you have about your feared situation? Make a list in your journal. Next, list possible strategies for getting your questions answered. Would it be most appropriate to talk to a dentist, doctor, or nurse about your concerns? Is there someone else you can ask? Can you find the information you're looking for on the Internet or at the library? Next, make an effort to get answers to your questions. Record what you learn in your journal.

challenging probability overestimations

One of the most common types of anxious thinking is often referred to as *probability overestimation*. Essentially, this involves overestimating the likelihood of something bad happening. Here are some examples of probability overestimation:

- ◊ I am definitely going to faint.

- ◊ The dentist will think I'm disgusting because I don't take care of my teeth.

- ◊ The doctor will tell me I have cancer.

- ◊ The needle will break off in my arm.

- ◊ The procedure will be very painful.

All of these statements are true for some people, some of the time. However, for people with phobias there's a tendency to assume these statements are true even when they're not, and to overestimate the likelihood of these events occurring. Replacing probability overestimations with more realistic predictions involves identifying your anxious belief, considering the evidence that supports your anxious belief, considering the evidence against your anxious belief, and settling on a more realistic belief, based on the evidence. Here's an example:

Anxious belief: I'll faint if I get a blood test.

Evidence in support of anxious belief: I fainted once about three years ago.

Evidence against anxious belief: I've had blood taken many times without fainting.

Rational conclusion: I may faint, but there's even a better chance that I won't.

If you have a history of frequent fainting (for example, fainting every time you have blood taken), this particular example may not apply to you. Remember, probability overestimations involve overestimating the likelihood of something happening. If you do tend to faint during most blood tests, predicting that you'll faint is not an overestimation. Rather, it is a realistic prediction. For such cases, it may be better to use strategies for combating catastrophic thinking, which we'll discuss shortly, as well as using the exposure and applied tension exercises reviewed in chapters 5 and 6.

---

exercise: examining the evidence

In your journal, record evidence for and against the anxious predictions you identified earlier in this chapter. Are your predictions necessarily true? What else might happen? What does your past experience tell you about what is most likely to happen? Are there other types of evidence (for example, information from your doctor or dentist) that you can include as you review the evidence for and against your anxious predictions? How might someone without anxiety think about this situation? Based on the evidence, what is a more realistic way of thinking about the situation? Once you've challenged your anxious prediction by reviewing the evidence, rate how strongly you now believe in the original anxious thought. Use the same scale ranging from 0 to 100, where 0 means you don't believe the prediction at all and 100 means you completely (or 100 percent) believe the prediction will come true. Did your rating change as a result of considering the evidence?

conquering catastrophic thinking

Catastrophic thinking involves overestimating how bad a particular outcome would be if it were to occur. People with phobias often assume that if their fear were to come true, it would be completely unmanageable, when in fact the situation is usually not as bad as they assume. If you find yourself using terms such as "unbearable," "overwhelming," and "terrible" to describe what would happen if you were to encounter your feared situation, ask yourself, "Would most people see this situation in the same way I do?" If not, it's possible that you're engaging in catastrophic thinking.

Challenging catastrophic thinking involves trying to put the situation in perspective by asking yourself questions such as these: What if my feared prediction were to come true? So what? Would it really matter, in the big scheme of things? Would it still matter tomorrow? How about the day after tomorrow? Next week? Rather than assuming the outcome would be unmanageable, ask your-self how you might cope with the situation if your predic-tion were to actually come true.

Here are some examples of common catastrophic thoughts concerning blood, needles, doctors, and den-tists, as well as examples of rational responses to these thoughts:

Catastrophic thought: It would be terrible if I were to faint.

Rational response: I've fainted before. It's uncomfortable, but usually I feel okay after about a half hour. The embar-rassment and discomfort would pass if I faint. If overcom-ing my fear through exposure means that I may faint a couple of times along the way, it's probably still worth it.

Catastrophic thought: The pain from the needle will be unbearable.

Rational response: Even if the pain is extreme, it will be over in a second or two. I can put up with almost anything for a second or two. Besides, just about everyone I know tells me that needles don't hurt.

Catastrophic thought: A visit to the dentist will be awful.

Rational response: People like me go to the dentist all the time, and they seem to survive. Chances are that I'll sur-vive as well. I need to remember that I have control over what happens at the dentist's. I can ask questions, and if there's a particular procedure I'm not ready for, I can always refuse to have it done.

Catastrophic thought: The anxiety I'd experience if I were to visit a hospital would be overwhelming.

Rational response: I've felt high levels of anxiety before, and I always manage to get through it. The worst thing that may happen is that I'll feel very uncomfortable. However, no matter how bad it is, the feeling will be temporary —the anxiety won't last forever. I can handle feeling uncomfortable for a short while.

exercise: challenging catastrophic thinking

In your journal, record any examples of catastrophic thinking that tend to arise when you think about confronting the situations you fear. Rate your anxiety about confronting your feared situation using a scale ranging from 0 to 100. Now, ask yourself a series of questions to challenge these thoughts: So what? Does it really matter whether my prediction comes true? What would the actual consequences be? Could I manage that? How could I cope with my prediction coming true? Try to answer these questions as realistically as possible. Now, once again rate your anxiety about confronting the feared situation. Did your anxiety level change as a result of challenging your catastrophic thinking?

troubleshooting

On their own, the cognitive strategies described in this chapter may not lead to significant reductions in your fear. But our intention is for you to use these strategies in combination with the exposure-based strategies described in chapter 5 (and the applied tension strategies described in chapter 6 if you have a history of fainting). With practice, you may find that the cognitive strategies help make your fear more manageable, allowing you to begin to confront your feared situations more easily.

The techniques described in this chapter may seem simple enough on the surface, but they are often quite difficult to use, particularly at the start. Two obstacles that often arise are difficulty identifying specific thoughts and difficulty believing the realistic thoughts you generate when challenging your anxious thoughts.

inability to identify specific thoughts

As mentioned earlier, the thoughts that contribute to fear and anxiety are often very automatic and quick, and may occur outside of awareness. Therefore, it may be difficult to identify specific negative predictions when you feel uncomfortable or anxious. If this is the case, we recommend that you continue to work on identifying your negative predictions. With practice, you may find it becomes easier. Consider the examples of anxious thoughts provided throughout this chapter. Do any of these seem to reflect what goes through your mind when you're anxious?

For some people, anxious predictions may be in the form of an image rather than a thought. Are you aware of any negative imagery concerning your feared situation? If so, what do you visualize happening when you imagine confronting the situation? If you have difficulty identifying thoughts and images concerning your feared situation, another strategy is to try to bring these on through exposure to the situation. Sometimes it's easier to identify your negative predictions when you're actually in the situation.

If all of these suggestions fail, there's still hope. Remember, the treatment of choice for fears of blood, needles, doctors, and dentists is repeated exposure to the situation. Fortunately, exposure is likely to be effective regardless of whether you're aware of the thoughts that contribute to your fear.

difficulty believing the rational thoughts

You may find that your anxious thoughts are so strong that it's difficult to believe the alternative, rational thoughts. Or, you may discover that generating alternatives to your anxious predictions doesn't lead to a reduction in your anxiety. For example, you may find yourself saying, "I know rationally that needles don't hurt, yet it's hard for me to believe that when I'm feeling anxious."

At first, trying to think realistically about the situation you fear may seem superficial. Even so, we recommend that you stick with it. You may find that, over time, your belief in the realistic alternatives strengthens and your belief in the anxious thoughts weakens. If your fear doesn't decrease even with practice, it may be that you're not considering all of the evidence. Perhaps there's additional information you should consider. If all else fails, don't worry. As we've mentioned, exposure is the most effective way to reduce your fear. If the cognitive strategies aren't helpful, focus more on your exposure practices until you overcome your fear.

summary

Anxiety is triggered by perceptions that a situation is dangerous or threatening. Identifying negative predictions about encountering blood, needles, doctors, and dentists and replacing them with more realistic beliefs is a useful way to combat anxiety and fear. This chapter reviewed particular types of anxious beliefs (probability overestimations and catastrophic thinking) and offered strategies for learning to think more realistically about the situations you fear.

8

staying well

Once treatment is over, how do you make sure your fear won't return? It's only natural that when you work hard at something, you want your gains to be maintained. While most people who use the steps in this book to overcome their fears will do quite well over the long term, there are some factors that may increase the likelihood of your fear reemerging after treatment has ended. It's important to make yourself aware of these potential pitfalls so that you can recognize and combat them if needed:

- ◊ Doing too little exposure after treatment has ended

- ◊ Returning to old habits of avoidance

- ◊ Experiencing increased life stress (for example, being under a deadline at work, experiencing conflict in a personal relationship, or having to cope with news of a serious illness of a good friend or relative)

◊ Confronting a new situation not previously faced on your exposure hierarchy

◊ Having a traumatic experience during an exposure

◊ Having an unexpected fear reaction during an exposure

We'll discuss each of these pitfalls and also provide some tips on dealing with each one so as to minimize the possibility of your fear returning.

doing too little exposure after treatment has ended

As you learned in chapter 5, the more frequently you practice exposure to your feared situations, the more effectively it will treat your phobia. The same is true over the long term. It's important that you continue to expose yourself to the feared object or situation occasionally, even after you're better. Look for everyday opportunities to continue to face your phobia. For example, if you were afraid of blood, seek out TV shows with surgical themes. If you had a fear of dentists, make sure you have regular dental checkups. You can even look for opportunities to accompany family members on dental visits. If your fear was directed toward needles or injections, become a regular blood donor. If you feared medical settings, look for opportunities to visit or even volunteer in a hospital.

Hang on to some of the exposure items you used to overcome your fear, such as videotapes, pictures, Web sites, needles, syringes, alcohol swabs, or anything else you used during your exposure exercises. Continue to expose yourself to these things on a regular basis. Figure out ways to have these items become a part of your everyday life. You might consider putting a screen saver of a feared image on your computer at home or at work. Put up pictures of feared images or place feared objects around your home in plain sight so that they become a part of your day-to-day life. Carry a feared object or image in your purse or briefcase or keep one in your drawer at work. Ongoing exposures like these should help maintain the gains you made earlier. Seek out these opportunities.

returning to old habits of avoidance

Closely related to the topic of inadequate exposure practices is the topic of increased avoidance. Before treatment, avoidance of certain feared situations or objects was probably common for you. You may have become so used to avoiding that you didn't recognize it when it was happening. When treatment of your phobia ends, it's important to ensure that you don't slip back into old patterns of avoidance. In particular, you need to be alert to the subtle ways avoidance can start to creep back into your life. Minor avoidance of fearful situations may make your day-to-day life a little less stressful, but you now know that this short-term relief will result in more anxiety over the long term. Small instances of avoidance can grow into larger ones, and avoidance strengthens fear. You may start to put off medical checkups or dental visits without really thinking about it. You may start to make excuses to get out of visiting a friend in the hospital. You may put off a blood test, flu shot, or other vaccination. Be on the lookout for minor instances of avoidance and address them right away, before they become larger.

You also need to be on the lookout for "avoidance by proxy." By that, we mean that well-intentioned family members and friends may have become accustomed to your fear over the years and may even be used to doing things for you in an attempt to help you avoid feeling uncomfortable. This may be so automatic that you and they may not even be aware of it. For example, they may avoid renting movies with violent scenes. Perhaps they warn you of fearful images in magazines you're planning to read. Or your spouse may offer to take the kids to the dentist when checkup time rolls around, instead of you. All of these are examples of subtle ways that others may make it easier for you to avoid your fears.

These well-intentioned but not so helpful acts need to be stopped when identified. For example, ask your friends and family to stop warning you about images or items that they worry might scare you. If you're fearful of blood, ask them to stop buying the meat at the butcher counter and offer to do it yourself. If you're afraid of needles, ask them to include you in the community blood donor drive. If you fear medical situations, ask them to stop avoiding conversations on medical topics when you're around. Every opportunity you can find to confront your phobia means that your phobia will become that much weaker.

experiencing increased life stress

We know that stress can strengthen fear. Life stresses such as marital conflict, job pressures, financial problems, or parenting pressures can increase your baseline level of anxiety. In other words, you may find that under stress you feel more on edge in general. In turn, a situation that would provoke a minimal fear response at times of low stress could cause a much more intense fear response at times of high stress. If you find that your fear seems to be returning, survey your life for any possible stresses. Work on reducing those stresses as much as possible. Look for ways to relax through such activities as exercise, meditation, listening to quiet music, or talking to a good friend. These are all great ways of managing those day-to-day stresses that can build up. Also, keep in mind that during stressful times you may have to increase the frequency of your exposures to counterbalance the negative effect of the stress. Luckily, once the life stress subsides, your fear will probably return to its prestress level.

confronting new situations

Suppose you successfully conquered your fear of needles by handling needles, watching needle-related videos, watching a friend have a vaccination, and eventually having a vaccination yourself. You may have gotten to the point of having very little anxiety in all the practice situations you confronted, and it may seem that you are completely over your fear of needles. But imagine that one day your doctor notices a mole that needs removal. You know this will involve use of a small scalpel followed by a few stitches—something that hadn't been a part of your initial exposure hierarchy. You might find that this new needle-related situation causes a lot of anxiety. It may feel that you're right back where you started, and this can be discouraging.

If this happens, just treat the new situation as another exposure exercise. Think of ways the exposure could be broken down into a mini hierarchy. Think of the various objects or situations you could expose yourself to as you confront this new fear. Begin to expose yourself to this new situation using the same methods as in chapter 5. Review the cognitive challenges you wrote about in your journal when working through the exercises in chapter 7. The great thing about exposure therapy is that once you understand the basics of it, it can be applied to almost any feared situation. Remember, you have all the tools to treat any new fear that arises. Have confidence in your new set of skills.

If you find that new, fearful situations emerge frequently, it might be a good idea to review your initial exposure hierarchy to make certain that it was as complete as you could make it. Make sure it was as varied as possible and that you tackled all of the steps on your hierarchy. Sometimes, as people approach their more difficult hierarchy steps, they seem to convince themselves that they've come far enough and don't really need to go any further. In fact, the further you can push yourself, the better off you'll be. Overshooting "normal" is a great goal to have. By this we mean that exposing yourself to situations that might cause anxiety even in people without phobias can give you a good buffer (especially if you experience any slight regressions in your improvement), as well as a great sense of accomplishment and the confidence to face any future challenges that arise.

having a traumatic experience during an exposure

Fear can sometimes return if you experience a traumatic event connected to one of your phobic situations. For example, let's suppose you conquered your fear of needles but later find yourself having blood drawn by an inexperienced lab technician who has to make five attempts to get the needle into your vein, causing a lot of distress and pain. Your fear of needles may be rekindled, and your initial impulse may be to start avoiding needles again. In this case, you need to remind yourself that avoidance will only serve to strengthen your fear. It's essential that you make every attempt to get back into the situation as soon as possible. If it's too difficult to return to that exact situation, look at your hierarchy and begin practicing in situations that are more manageable. Remember, you have all the tools you need to treat this fear before it gets out of hand.

Reacting with fear during a traumatic incident is common and to be expected even in people without a preexisting phobia. Don't get discouraged.

having an unexpected fear reaction during an exposure

Imagine that you worked your way up your exposure hierarchy to overcome your fear of dentists. You arranged to have some dental work done over four different appointments in order to give yourself frequent exposure opportunities. The first three appointments went well and you've managed your anxiety successfully. You then go to your fourth appointment and, for whatever reason (maybe you skipped breakfast that morning, or perhaps you're out of breath from taking the stairs instead of the elevator), you begin to feel faint in the chair. You're feeling short of breath and you worry you'll pass out. Your anxiety increases, and you start to experience a panic attack in the dentist's chair. This is all quite unexpected, because everything had gone so smoothly up to this point. Such an experience might serve to rekindle your fear if you're not careful.

Unexpected reactions can happen during exposures, whether they're planned exposures (as part of your hierarchy) or exposures that occur as part of your everyday life. These reactions don't mean that your treatment isn't working or that you're back where you started. A return of some anxiety symptoms in such a case is normal and expected. Trust that all your hard work to this point will see you through and don't get discouraged. It's important that you continue with your exposure practices right away. The longer you wait to return to your exposures, the more difficult it will be. If you find that fainting-related symptoms begin to reemerge in situations you thought you had conquered, you may need to review your applied tension exercises (chapter 6) and reintroduce applied tension into some of your exposures for the short term.

exercise: identifying your potential pitfalls

In your journal, write out a list of potential factors that may increase the likelihood of your fear returning. Use the information in this chapter as a starting point to help construct your list. Next to each potential obstacle on your list, write out a potential solution, including the suggestions mentioned in this chapter, as well as any other solutions you can think of. Do you have a tendency to stop doing exposures once you feel you're better? If so, how can you make exposures part of your life? Are there people in your life who unintentionally still help you avoid challenging situations? If so, how will you address this with them? Are there potential life stresses that can be managed or eliminated? How will you do this? Did you include enough exposures on your hierarchy initially, and did you confront every situation that you intended to confront? If not, how can your hierarchy be modified? How will you handle new situations that you hadn't previously even considered?

What will you do if you have an unexpected fear reaction in an exposure situation? For those who tend to faint, are your applied tension skills second nature, or do they need to be reviewed?

some final words on judging your progress fairly

Sometimes people become discouraged during treatment if they experience minor worsening of symptoms along the way. It's important to remember that improvement usually doesn't occur in a straight line. In other words, each new day is not necessarily better than the preceding day. Other areas of life are like this as well. Take, for example, athletic performance. Suppose you're learning to run and you've entered yourself in a five-mile race two months from now. You sign up for a sixty-day "Learn to Run Five Miles" training program at your local gym. In training for that race, you'll find that some days you feel better and can run faster than on other days. There's no guarantee that you'll run faster on day five of your training schedule than you did on day one. You may actually run more slowly because of normal day-to-day variance. In fact, if you compare your performance on day one to your performance on day five and use just that measurement as your gauge of progress, you might think your running skills are worsening rather than improving. But what if you compare day one with day sixty? Chances are that your running will be better on day sixty of your training program than it was on day one.

When you measure improvement, it's important to use an appropriate time interval for comparison. If the intervals are too close together (like day one and day five), it may seem as though you're making no progress or, even worse, that you're regressing. Considering your progress over such a short time interval doesn't take into account life's normal ups and downs, and it may not provide an accurate reflection of longer-term improvement. Don't fall into this trap as you work on conquering your fears. There will be normal ups and downs as you progress through treatment. There will be normal ups and downs even after treatment. If you focus on these day-to-day variations, you may become discouraged and may even stop treatment early, all based on an unfair evaluation of your progress. Expect some normal ups and downs as you work on conquering your fear. It's the long-term picture that really matters.

summary

A number of factors can compromise the long-term effectiveness of exposure therapy. These factors include avoidance, infrequent opportunities for exposure, life stresses, confronting new situations, and having a traumatic experience or an unexpected fear reaction during an exposure. The impact of these pitfalls can be minimized if you recognize the problem early on and follow up with a helpful action plan aimed at overcoming these obstacles. This will lay the groundwork for continued long-term well-being. Occasional ups and downs during treatment and even after treatment are normal and shouldn't discourage you from continuing with what you started.

9

for the helper

If you've been asked to read this chapter, it means that you've agreed to help a person you know overcome a medical phobia. The person's decision to work on overcoming this fear may have been a difficult one to make. In doing so, that person knows there's a risk of increased anxiety and discomfort in the short term in return for long-term freedom from the phobia. It's important that you read this chapter, where we'll outline some basic rules to help you be the most effective helper you can be. It's also important that you read the rest of the book so that you have a thorough understanding of what's involved in conquering a fear. A large part of the treatment's success lies with you, and we want to give you the tools and guidance you need to help maximize this success.

be empathic

One of the most important tools for a helper to have is empathy—the ability to imagine what another person is experiencing emotionally. In helping someone face a fear, it's helpful if you can imagine that person's level of discomfort when faced with a phobic object or situation. Often, this may be difficult to do, especially if you don't share that person's fear. No matter how trivial or ridiculous the fear may seem to you, you must try to understand the person's experience as well as you can. Try to think of something that frightens you. Now try to imagine how you'd feel if you deliberately exposed yourself to that situation day after day. That's how the phobic person feels in this treatment program. Don't trivialize the fear, and don't ridicule the individual. For the person you're helping, the emotions are very real even if the anticipated danger is exaggerated. Be supportive. Recognize the individual's courage in facing his or her fear.

no surprises allowed

Exposure therapy must be completely within the control of the person being treated. That means he or she decides what exposures will be done, when they will be done, and how long they'll last. Exposures are supposed to be predictable, which means that surprising a person with a feared object is not allowed, no matter how well-intentioned the action is. The person you're helping should know ahead of time everything that will happen during the exposure practice.

be supportive

The process of conquering a phobia can be exhausting, challenging, and filled with ups and downs. It's not unusual for a person confronting a fear to become discouraged from time to time. An exposure exercise that didn't go so well, an unexpected fear reaction, or a slow course of improvement can take a toll on the positive attitude of the person. You should be there to give words of encouragement and point out the successes along the way. You should maintain an objective point of view and help the person remember the reasons for doing this, especially when things seem tough. If, as a helper, you become discouraged during the rough patches, try not to let it show and try not to let it affect your outward display of a positive attitude.

be encouraging (but not pushy)

Sometimes the difference between being encouraging and being pushy is a fine line to walk. As a helper, you should gently encourage the person who is facing a fear to push himself or herself to the limit, but you should never force the person to stay in a situation, hold an object, or watch an image longer than he or she has agreed to. Some people need more encouragement than others. Ask the person you're working with how you can best provide encourage-ment to stay with an exposure if the fear becomes intense. Ask what words of encouragement you can provide. The individual should know best what style of support he or she finds most motivating.

screen exposure items ahead of time

Before exposure can begin, a number of exposure-related objects or situations need to be located (see chapter 4). Because these may cause extreme anxiety for the person being treated (especially at the start of treatment), you may have to prescreen some of the items to determine their suitability for exposure at various stages of the treat-ment. You may want to describe an image or a situation rather than show it to the person and have him or her decide what fear ranking to assign to that object or situa-tion based on your description. You can also help brain-storm various exposure possibilities.

demonstrate a positive coping strategy

During the actual exposure exercises, it can be helpful for you to do the exposure yourself first, while the person you're helping looks on. For example, if you're helping someone with a fear of blood, you may prick your finger with a lancet while he or she watches. This will accom-plish two things. First, watching the situation will be an exposure in itself. Second, watching you confront the situ-ation in a controlled, safe way will help model a positive response and will educate the person about the real danger of the situation versus his or her belief about the degree of danger. It's often easier to do something frightening if we watch someone we trust do it first.

Before modeling a positive coping style, though, you need to make sure you don't have a fear of the object or situation yourself, so you can guarantee that your reaction won't be anxiety provoking. You may want to expose yourself to the object or situation ahead of time, in the absence of the person you're helping. If you find you do have some minor fear, you might consider engaging in a few repeated exposure exercises yourself, before helping the person with the phobia.

help challenge anxiety-provoking thoughts

The fear that people experience during exposure exercises is a direct result of what they're thinking before or during the exercise (see chapter 7). Therefore, it can be beneficial for you to help the phobic person monitor any thoughts that occur before and during the exposure. Help challenge unrealistic or exaggerated negative beliefs or predictions using the strategies described in chapter 7. For example, during an exposure exercise, you may want to ask such questions as "What are you thinking right now?" "How likely is it that your feared outcome will happen?" "If your feared outcome (for example, fainting) were to happen, how would you cope?" "What evidence do you have that your negative predictions are true?" These questions will help the person see the situation more realistically and less catastrophically.

respect confidentiality

When you engage in a therapeutic relationship with a person for treatment of a phobia, you must respect that person's right to have anything that goes on in treatment to remain between the two of you. Don't tell other family members or friends about the treatment or about the details of the person's phobia (unless the person you're helping gives clear permission to do so).

be dependable

If you commit to helping a person overcome a fear, you must take that commitment seriously. That means being dependable. Be on time for exposure exercises. Follow through on promises made. If you commit to helping out on a certain day, don't cancel at the last minute. The person you're helping has to know you'll be there. He or she has made a commitment to get over the fear and is relying on you to help. Your commitment needs to be just as strong.

make it enjoyable

People are more likely to continue with an activity if it's enjoyable. Although exposure is usually anxiety provoking and the work may be quite difficult at times, anything you can do to make things more enjoyable will go a long way toward enhancing the treatment. Have a positive attitude and maintain a sense of humor. Try to be upbeat. Share in the successes of the patient. Plan a reward for a job well done (for example, a dinner out or a movie). When helping to design exposure practices, use your imagination to make the process as exciting, adventurous, and fun as possible.

be prepared for minor setbacks

Sometimes treatment proceeds smoothly, with very few hiccups along the way. But other times, there may be set-backs. Don't become discouraged. If a particular practice is too difficult, you can help the individual review the hierarchy and come up with items that may be more suit-able. Remind the person that the road to success is full of ups and downs and reinforce the idea that you'll be there through those highs and lows. Encourage the individual to have confidence that the hard work will pay off in the end.

help with fainting

Although fainting is very rare in other types of phobias (for example, phobias of animals, heights, driving, and fly-ing), people who fear blood and needles often faint during exposure to the objects and situations they fear (see chap-ter 6). Therefore, it's possible that the person you're help-ing will faint during an exposure. Don't panic. If fainting is a risk with the person you're helping, make sure you dis-cuss it ahead of time so you can provide reassurance that you'll be there to help in case he or she faints. Prior to an exposure exercise, ask the person to describe his or her usual early warning signs of an oncoming faint so you know what to watch for. During the exercise, have the person let you know if any of these symptoms occur, so you can be prepared to help.

If the person does faint, try to break the fall by catching the individual and gently laying him or her in a horizontal position, preferably on the side. Raising the person's legs slightly may help speed recovery from the fainting episode. Be calm. Most people recover from a faint within seconds. You should also review the applied tension exercises discussed in chapter 6 so that you can remind the person you're helping to put these into practice when needed.

know what to say during an exposure exercise

Knowing exactly what to say during an actual exposure practice can be a challenge. Words of encouragement, such as "Good job," "Stick with it; you're doing fine," or "Look how far you've come" are usually helpful.

Helping the person monitor his or her fear level can also be helpful. Ask the individual to provide a fear rating, based on a scale ranging from 0 to 100, at intervals throughout the exposure exercise. This will help both of you monitor the progress. It will also let you know when you might move on to a more difficult hierarchy item. Once the fear rating falls below 60 or so, many people will be able to move on to a more difficult step on the hierarchy. A fear level of less than 30 is a sure sign to move to a more challenging practice. If the fear rating remains high, this is a sign to slow down, take your time, and wait for the fear to decrease before moving on to the next step on the hierarchy. For example, if the fear rating is between 60 and 80, it's probably best to continue with that particular step. A fear rating higher than 80 definitely signals that more time is needed before moving up the hierarchy. It's important for the person to try to stay in the fearful situation until the fear level clearly declines. Leaving the exposure while fear is high or on the rise may serve to reinforce avoidance, which will strengthen rather than weaken the fear.

example of a discussion during an exposure practice

Taking into account the points we have discussed so far, an exposure exercise for Aaron, who has a blood phobia, might go something like this:

Helper: Okay, now let's try watching a short videotape of a knee operation. *(Puts tape in VCR.)* How are you feeling right now, as you're about to watch this scene for the first time?

Aaron: I'm a little scared. I would rank my fear at about an 80, but I don't know how I'll react when I push the "play" button.

Helper: Okay, I'm here with you. So far so good. Go ahead and push the "play" button whenever you're ready.

Aaron: Alright, here goes. *(Pushes "play" and the scene starts.)* I'm nervous. My fear is rising. It's actually about a 90 now. I don't know if I can continue to watch this.

Helper: You're doing great. Hang in there if you can. Try not to look away. What are you thinking right now that makes your fear a 90?

Aaron: I don't know if I can watch the blood. I might lose control or freak out. Or, I may faint. It's disgusting.

Helper: You are watching it and you're doing fine. Do you really think you'll freak out? What do you think will realistically happen?

Aaron: Well, I guess at the very worst I'll be disgusted, and that's okay. I've dealt with being disgusted before. I may feel faint as well, but I know I can do applied tension and I know that you're here to help if I do faint. *(Continues to watch the video for another fifteen minutes.)*

Helper: How would you rate your anxiety now, as you continue to watch this scene?

Aaron: I think it's going down. I seem to be getting used to this scene. It's about a 70. *(Video ends.)*

Helper: You're doing great. I know this is tough for you, but you're doing just great. Let's watch that scene again and see if we can get that anxiety any lower.

Aaron: Okay. *(Presses "play" again.)* I'm not nearly so anxious this time. I would say I'm now at about a 40. Actually, this video is kind of interesting; disgusting, but interesting.

Helper: How would you feel about looking at a slightly more bloody video of a hip surgery?

Aaron: Let's try it.

As you can see, the helper gives lots of support, checks in on fear ratings, goes at an appropriate pace, allows Aaron to control the exposure, gently encourages Aaron not to avoid, helps combat inaccurate cognitions, and suggests further exposures.

summary

As a helper to someone attempting to combat his or her phobia, there are certain guidelines you should follow to be as successful as possible. Your attitude, your words of encouragement, and your support and dependability can make a big difference. In this chapter we reviewed some of the more important characteristics of a good helper and provided suggestions for how a helper can optimize the treatment experience. Helping a person conquer a phobia is a big responsibility for sure, but it can also be incredibly rewarding.

references

American Psychiatric Association. 1994. *Diagnostic and Statistical Manual of Mental Disorders*. 4th ed. Washington, D.C.: American Psychiatric Association.

Antony, M. M., and D. H. Barlow. 2002. Specific phobia. In *Anxiety and Its Disorders: The Nature and Treatment of Anxiety and Panic*, 2nd ed., edited by D. H. Barlow, 380–417. New York: Guilford Press.

Antony, M. M., T. A. Brown, and D. H. Barlow. 1997. Heterogeneity among specific phobia types in DSM-IV. *Behaviour Research and Therapy* 35:1089–1100.

Antony, M. M., and R. P. Swinson. 2000. *Phobic Disorders and Panic in Adults: A Guide to Assessment and Treatment*. Washington, DC: Amercian Psychological Association.

Asmundson, G. J. G., and S. Taylor. 2005. *It's Not All in Your Head: How Worrying About Your Health Could Be Making You Sick—and What You Can Do About It.* New York: Guilford Press.

Butcher, J. L., M. Hirai, L. Vernon, J. L. Stransky, H. M. Cochran, and E. A. Meadows. 2003. Assessing the efficacy of treatment targeting disgust and fear in blood and injection phobia. Paper presented at the meeting of the Association for Advancement of Behavior Therapy, Boston.

Curtis, G. C., W. J. Magee, W. W. Eaton, H.-U. Wittchen, and R. C. Kessler. 1998. Specific fears and phobias: Epidemiology and classification. *British Journal of Psychiatry* 173:212–217.

Davis, M., E. R. Eshelman, and M. McKay. 2000. *The Relaxation and Stress Reduction Workbook.* 5th ed. Oakland, Calif.: New Harbinger Publications.

de Jongh, A., P. Muris, G. T. Horst, F. van Zuuren, N. Schoenmakers, and P. Makkes. 1995. One session cognitive treatment of dental phobia: Preparing dental phobics for treatment by restructuring negative cognitions. *Behaviour Research and Therapy* 33:947–954.

Febrarro, G. A. R., G. A. Clum, A. A. Roodman, and J. H. Wright. 1999. The limits of bibliotherapy: A study of the differential effectiveness of self-administered interventions in individuals with panic attacks. *Behavior Therapy* 30:209222.

Fredrikson, M., P. Annas, H. Fischer, and G. Wik. 1996. Gender and age differences in the prevalence of specific fears and phobias. *Behaviour Research and Therapy* 26:241–244.

Getka, E. J., and C. R. Glass. 1992. Behavioral and cognitive-behavioral approaches to the reduction of dental anxiety. *Behavior Therapy* 23:433–448.

Glassner, B. 1999. *The Culture of Fear: Why Americans Are Afraid of the Wrong Things.* New York: Basic Books.

Gould, R. A., and G. A. Clum. 1995. Self-help plus minimal therapist contact in the treatment of panic disorder: A replication and extension. *Behavior Therapy* 26:533–546.

Heckscher, M. 2004. *Be Safe! Simple Strategies for Death-Free Living.* Philadelphia: Quirk Books.

Hellström, K., J. Fellenius, and L.-G. Öst. 1996. One versus five sessions of applied tension in the treatment of blood phobia. *Behaviour Research and Therapy* 34:101–112.

Hellström, K., and L.-G. Öst. 1995. One-session therapist directed exposure vs. two forms of manual directed self-exposure in the treatment of spider phobia. *Behaviour Research and Therapy* 33:959–965.

Hettema, J. M., M. C. Neale, and K. S. Kendler. 2001. A review and meta-analysis of the genetic epidemiology of anxiety disorders. *American Journal of Psychiatry* 158:1568–1578.

Himle, J. A., K. McPhee, O. J. Cameron, and G. C. Curtis. 1989. Simple phobia: Evidence for heterogeneity. *Psychiatry Research* 28:25–30.

Jerremalm, A., L. Jansson, and L.-G. Öst. 1986. Individual response patterns and the effects of different behavioral methods in the treatment of dental phobia. *Behaviour Research and Therapy* 24:587–596.

Kendler, K. S., L. M. Karkowski, and C. A. Prescott. 1999. Fear and phobias: Reliability and heritability. *Psychological Medicine* 29:539–553.

Kendler, K. S., J. Myers, and C. A. Prescott. 2002. The etiology of phobias: An evaluation of the stress-diathesis model. *Archives of General Psychiatry* 59:242–248.

Kent, G. 1985. Cognitive processes in dental anxiety. *British Journal of Clinical Psychology* 24:259–264.

Kleinknecht, R. A. 1994. Acquisition of blood, injury, and needle fears and phobias. *Behaviour Research and Therapy* 32:817–823.

Kleinknecht, R. A., and J. Lenz. 1989. Blood/injury fear, fainting, and avoidance of medically related situations: A family correspondence study. *Behaviour Research and Therapy* 27:537–547.

Kozak, M. J., and G. A. Miller. 1985. The psychophysiological process of therapy in a case of injury-scene-elicited fainting. *Journal of Behavior Therapy and Experimental Psychiatry* 16:139–145.

Kozak, M. J., and G. K. Montgomery. 1981. Multimodal behavioral treatment of recurrent injury-scene elicited fainting (vasodepressor syncope). *Behavioural Psychotherapy* 9:316–321.

Larson, K. H., G. Kvale, E. Skaret, E. Berg, M. Raadal, and L.-G. Öst. 2004. One-session treatment of dental phobia (DP): A randomized controlled trial. Paper presented at the meeting of the Association for Advancement of Behavior Therapy, New Orleans.

Lee, L. 2004. *100 Most Dangerous Things in Everyday Life and What You Can Do About Them.* New York: Broadway Books.

Moore, R., and I. Brødsgaard. 1994. Group therapy compared with individual desensitization for dental anxiety. *Community Dentistry and Oral Epidemiology* 22:258–262.

Neale, M. C., E. E. Walters, L. J. Eaves, R. C. Kessler, A. C. Heath, and K. S. Kendler. 1994. Genetics of blood-injury fears and phobias: A population-based twin study. *American Journal of Medical Genetics* 54:326–334.

Öst, L.-G. 1985. Ways of acquiring phobias and outcome of behavioural treatment. *Behaviour Research and Therapy* 23:683–689.

Öst, L.-G. 1987. Age of onset of different phobias. *Journal of Abnormal Psychology* 96:223–229.

Öst, L.-G. 1989. One-session treatment for specific phobias. *Behaviour Research and Therapy* 27:1–7.

Öst, L.-G. 1991. Acquisition of blood and injection phobia and anxiety response patterns in clinical patients. *Behaviour Research and Therapy* 29:323–332.

Öst, L.-G. 1992. Blood and injection phobia: Background and cognitive, physiological, and behavioral variables. *Journal of Abnormal Psychology* 101:68–74.

Öst, L.-G., J. Fellenius, and U. Sterner. 1991. Applied tension, exposure in vivo, and tension-only in the treatment of blood phobia. *Behaviour Research and Therapy* 29:561–574.

Öst, L.-G., and K. Hugdahl. 1985. Acquisition of blood and dental phobia and anxiety response patterns in clinical patients. *Behaviour Research and Therapy* 23:27–34.

Öst, L.-G., and U. Sterner. 1987. Applied tension: A specific behavioral method for treatment of blood phobia. *Behaviour Research and Therapy* 25:25–29.

Öst, L.-G., U. Sterner, and J. Fellenius. 1989. Applied tension, applied relaxation, and the combination in the treatment of blood phobia. *Behaviour Research and Therapy* 27:109–121.

Öst, L.-G., U. Sterner, and I.-L. Lindahl. 1984. Physiological responses in blood phobics. *Behaviour Research and Therapy* 22:109–117.

Öst, L.-G., B.-M. Stridh, and M. Wolf. 1998. A clinical study of spider phobia: Prediction of outcome after self-help and therapist-directed treatments. *Behaviour Research and Therapy* 36:17–35.

Page, A. C. 1994. Blood-injury phobia. *Clinical Psychology Review* 14:443–461.

Page, A. C., and N. G. Martin. 1998. Testing a genetic structure of blood-injury-injection fears. *American Journal of Medical Genetics* 81:377–384.

Panzarella, C., and J. Garlipp. 1999. Integration of cognitive techniques into an individualized application of behavioral treatment of blood-injection-injury phobia. *Cognitive and Behavioral Practice* 6:200–211.

Park, J.-M., D. Mataix-Cols, I. M. Marks, T. Ngamthipwatthana, M. Marks, R. Araya, and T. Al-Kubaisy. 2001. Two-year follow-up after a randomised controlled trial of self- and clinician-accompanied exposure for phobia/panic disorders. *British Journal of Psychiatry* 178:543–548.

Poulton, R., W. M. Thomson, R. H. Brown, and P. A. Silva. 1998. Dental fear with and without blood-injection fear: Implications for dental health and clinical practice. *Behaviour Research and Therapy* 36:591–597.

Rachman, S. 1977. The conditioning theory of fear-acquisition: A critical examination. *Behaviour Research and Therapy* 15:375–387.

Ropeik, D., and G. Gray. 2002. *Risk! A Practical Guide for Deciding What's Really Safe and What's Really Dangerous in the World Around You.* Boston: Houghton Mifflin.

Sawchuk, C. N., T. C. Lee, D. F. Tolin, and J. M. Lohr. 1997. Generalized disgust sensitivity in blood-injection-injury phobia. Paper presented at the meeting of the Association for Advancement of Behavior Therapy, Miami Beach.

Schwartz, S. G., P. S. J. Adler, and D. G. Kaloupek. 1987. Sources of variation in human fear responding: Subtypes, cue content, and coping. Paper presented at the meeting of the Association for Advancement of Behavior Therapy, Boston.

Skre, I., S. Onstad, O. S. Torgerson, S. Lygren, and E. Kringlen. 1993. A twin study of DSM-III-R anxiety disorders. *Acta Psychiatrica Scandinavica* 88:85–92.

Thom, A., G. Sartory, and P. Jöhren. 2000. Comparison between one-session psychological treatment and benzodiazepine in dental phobia. *Journal of Consulting and Clinical Psychology* 68:378–387.

Thompson, A. 1999. Cognitive-behavioural treatment of blood-injury-injection phobia: A case study. *Behaviour Change* 16:182–190.

Tolin, D. F., J. M. Lohr, C. N. Sawchuk, and T. C. Lee. 1997. Disgust and disgust sensitivity in blood-injection-injury and spider phobia. *Behaviour Research and Therapy* 35:949–953.

Townend, E., G. Dimigen, and D. Fung. 2000. A clinical study of child dental anxiety. *Behaviour Research and Therapy* 38:31–46.

Woody, S. R., and B. A. Teachman. 2000. Intersection of disgust and fear: Normative and pathological views. *Clinical Psychology: Science and Practice* 7:291–311.

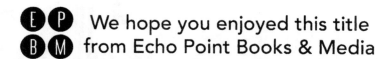

We hope you enjoyed this title
from Echo Point Books & Media

Before Closing this Book, Two Good Things to Know

Buy Direct & Save

Go to www.echopointbooks.com (click "Our Titles" at top or click "For Echo Point Publishing" in the middle) to see our complete list of titles. We publish books on a wide variety of topics—from spirituality to auto repair.

Buy direct and save 10% at www.echopointbooks.com

DISCOUNT CODE: EPBUYER

Make Literary History and Earn $100 Plus Other Goodies Simply for Your Book Recommendation!

At Echo Point Books & Media we specialize in republishing out-of-print books that are united by one essential ingredient: high quality. Do you know of any great books that are no longer actively published? If so, please let us know. If we end up publishing your recommendation, you'll be adding a wee bit to literary culture and a bunch to our publishing efforts.

Here is how we will thank you:

- A free copy of the new version of your beloved book that includes acknowledgement of your skill as a sharp book scout.
- A free copy of another Echo Point title you like from echopointbooks.com.
- And, oh yes, we'll also send you a check for $100.

Since we publish an eclectic list of titles, we're interested in a wide range of books. So please don't be shy if you have obscure tastes or like books with a practical focus. To get a sense of what kind of books we publish, visit us at www.echopointbooks.com.

If you have a book that you think will work for us, send us an email at editorial@echopointbooks.com

CPSIA information can be obtained
at www.ICGtesting.com
Printed in the USA
BVHW080901070121
597128BV00003B/158

9 781626 543515